WAY

BREATHW⬤RKS FOR YOUR BACK

FUNDS TO PURCHASE
THIS BOOK WERE
PROVIDED BY A
40TH ANNIVERSARY GRANT
FROM THE
FOELLINGER FOUNDATION.

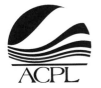

ACPL

✓

BREATHW**FOR YOUR BACK**ORKS

STRENGTHENING YOUR BACK FROM THE INSIDE OUT

NANCY SWAYZEE, MES, CHFI

AVON BOOKS ◆ NEW YORK

Every effort has been made in this book's preparation to stress the need for proper technique and body alignment. Before beginning any exercise program, however, check with your healthcare practitioner to make sure it is appropriate for you. While you're on this, or any, exercise program, it is advisable to visit your physician or healthcare practitioner for periodic monitoring. It is suggested that you read through the text once to become familiar with the exercises before beginning the program. Follow all instructions carefully and do not do any exercise or stretch that causes pain or discomfort. Not all exercises are suitable for everyone. The instructions and advice are in no way intended as a substitute for medical counseling.

Medical illustrations on pages 20, 22, 23 are from *Muscles: Testing and Function, Fourth Edition.* Copyright © 1993 by Williams & Wilkins. Used by permission.

PEANUTS cartoon reprinted by permission of United Features Syndicate, Inc.

AVON BOOKS
A division of
The Hearst Corporation
1350 Avenue of the Americas
New York, New York 10019

Copyright © 1998 by Nancy Swayzee
Illustrations by Janice Polucha
Interior design by Rhea Braunstein
Published by arrangement with the author
Visit our website at **http://www.AvonBooks.com**
ISBN: 0-380-79044-0

Library of Congress Cataloging in Publication Data:
Swayzee, Nancy L.
Breathworks for your back : strengthening your back from the inside out / by Nancy L. Swayzee.
p.   cm.
Includes bibliographical references.
1. Backache—Exercise therapy   2. Abdominal exercises.
3. Back—Care and hygiene.   I. Title.
RD771.B217S93   1998   97-36517
617.5'64062—dc21   CIP

First Avon Books Trade Printing: April 1998

AVON TRADEMARK REG. U.S. PAT. OFF. AND IN OTHER COUNTRIES, MARCA REGISTRADA, HECHO EN U.S.A.

Printed in the U.S.A.

OPM   10 9 8 7 6 5 4 3 2 1

This book is dedicated to my children, Michael and Lori; to Kristy, my daughter through marriage; and to the two bright stars in my universe, Madeline and Mason.

Through the creation of this book I express my wonder and gratitude for the gifts the universe has given me.

ACKNOWLEDGMENTS

My everlasting gratitude to my friend, adviser, consultant, and playmate, Peggy Ricketts, for her hours of patient guidance as I struggled to understand my computer; for her repeated rereading, retesting, and reentering the material to ensure that it was clear; for her unwavering persistence that I modify, simplify, and cut; and for her brilliant organizational skills, which allowed this project to reach completion.

Deep and sincere appreciation to my editor, Lisa Considine, who approached every word with thoughtful questioning, playing devil's advocate, and suggested changes that clarified and polished my first draft of the manuscript.

To Gareth Ersersky, my agent, whose belief in this project is what took the book from just a dream into actual publication.

My thanks to David Spilver, who was patient, supportive, and realistic in his guidance during the first three years of this undertaking.

My deep gratitude to Laurel Hilde and Tom Lippert, who started this project with me, and performed their editorial and photographic skills without the benefit of immediate compensation.

And to Ben, for his creative suggestions and insights, for pushing me to work when I wanted to play, and for his continuous support, encouragement, and love.

A special thanks to Michael McQuarrie, M.D., F.A.C.E.P., for his belief in the worthiness of this project and for his unsolicited assistance and support in my efforts to interest the physician staff at Tahoe Forest Hospital.

To Richard Gepford, P.T. for his encouragement, support, and valuable advice.

A loving "thank you" to Janet Brady, for her faith in my ability and my vision and for the opportunity to reach the medical community and introduce this program through Tahoe Forest Hospital.

Last, and with immeasurable appreciation to the people who inspired the creation of this book, Lori Myers, R.P.T., who not only played a major role in the rehabilitation of my back after my injury, but also for her role as consultant and adviser in the beginning development of the abdominal exercises; for introducing me to the text that was to change my life: *Muscles: Testing and Function,* by Florence P. Kendall and Elizabeth Kendall McCreary.

Without the simplicity and clarity of the text and the illustrations in this book, the original concept of using forced expiration of breath might never have happened.

CONTENTS

Introduction   1

1: Getting to the Core of the Matter   13

PART I Abdominal Strengthening Program   41

2: Basic Training (Or Exercise That Doesn't
   Feel Like Exercise)   43
3: Passive Resistance   60
4: Crunching the Numbers   85

PART II Range of Motion Exercises   101

5: Within Range   103
6: Getting to the Bottom of Things   127

PART III Back-Strengthening Program   149

7: Back to Back Basics   151

PART IV Stretching Program 191

8: Moving into the Home Stretch 193
9: Standing Up for Yourself 225
10: Wrapping It Up 240

Bibliography 247

EXERCISES

Exercise 1. Belly-Breathing   45
Exercise 2. Active Belly Breathing   46
Exercise 3. Basic Supine In and Up   48
Exercise 4. In and Up on Hands and Knees   51
Exercise 5. Standing Forced Expiration of Breath   54
Exercise 6. Butterfly Arm Move   61
Exercise 7. Angels in the Snow   63
Exercise 8. Alternate Arm Move   65
Exercise 9. Standing Alternate Arm Move   67
Exercise 10. Side-Lying Active In and Up   71
Exercise 11. Prone Active In and Up   72
Exercise 12. Double Heel Slides   74
Exercise 13. Extended Leg Movement   76
Exercise 14. Single Leg Lower and Lift   78
Exercise 15. Alternate Heel Slides   81
Exercise 16. Hands and Knees Diagonal Extension   82
Exercise 17. Hands and Knees with Pelvic Rotation   91
Exercise 18. Supine In and Up with Pelvic Rotation   92
Exercise 19. Side-Lying In and Up with Curl
             and Extension   94
Exercise 20. Alternate Arm and Leg Move   96
Exercise 21. Standing Oblique Crunch   97
Exercise 22. Alternate Arm Angels in the Snow   114
Exercise 23. Alternate Arm Sweep   115

Exercise 24. Opposite Hand to Arm Move   116
Exercise 25. Alternate Hand to Opposite Knee   117
Exercise 26. Side-Lying Arm Circles   119
Exercise 27. Side-Lying Elbow Circles   121
Exercise 28. Side-Lying Arm Slide   122
Exercise 29. Side-Lying Chest Stretch   124
Exercise 30. Bicycle Pump with External Rotation   132
Exercise 31. Standing Single-Leg Knee Bend   134
Exercise 32. Prone Gluteal Squeeze Lift   135
Exercise 33. Bridges   137
Exercise 34. Bench Squats   139
Exercise 35. Seated Gluteal Squeezes   140
Exercise 36. Double Bent-Knee Rolls   142
Exercise 37. Supine Pelvic Pump   144
Exercise 38. Single-Knee Roll-ins   145
Exercise 39. Double Bent-Knee Body Curl   147
Exercise 40. Bench-Seated Wall Press with Breath   163
Exercise 41. Bench-Seated Arm Raise with Breath   164
Exercise 42. Supine Shoulder Blade Squeeze   166
Exercise 43. Shoulder Blade Squeeze with External
             Arm Rotation   167
Exercise 44. Supine Butterfly Arm Pull-Down   168
Exercise 45. Double Bent-Knee Body Curl   170
Exercise 46. Prone Back Lift 1   171
Exercise 47. Prone Back Lift 2   172
Exercise 48. Prone Butterfly Arm Lift   173
Exercise 49. Prone Shoulder Blade Squeeze   175
Exercise 50. Prone Back Lift 3   176
Exercise 51. Cat Back Stretch Combo   177
Exercise 52. Wall Standing   178
Exercise 53. Seated C Curl-up   180
Exercise 54. Standing Roll-up Shoulder Shrug   181
Exercise 55. Overhead Wall Press   183
Exercise 56. Wide-Arm Wall Press   184
Exercise 57. Wall Push-up   185
Exercise 58. Standing 90-Degree External Arm
             Rotation   186
Exercise 59. Double Bent-Knee Body Rolls with
             Angels in the Snow   200

Exercise 60. Single-Knee Roll-ins with Angels in
the Snow 203
Exercise 61. Supine Pelvic Pump 204
Exercise 62. Double Bent-Knee Body Curl 205
Exercise 63. Back-Lying Hip Stretch 205
Exercise 64. Single Knee to Chest 207
Exercise 65. Side-Lying Pelvic Pump 208
Exercise 66. Side-Lying Upper Back and
Chest Stretch 209
Exercise 67. Side-Lying Curl and Extension 212
Exercise 68. Prone Diagonal Extension 213
Exercise 69. Cat Back Stretch Combo 214
Exercise 70. Prayer Position Back and Chest Stretch 215
Exercise 71. Extended Abdominal and Hip
Flexor Stretch 216
Exercise 72. Hands and Knees Diagonal Extension 217
Exercise 73. Lowering Bridge Stretch 219
Exercise 74. Single Knee-to-Chest Curl and Extension 220
Exercise 75. Full Supine Starfish Extension 221
Exercise 76. Standing Calf Stretch 227
Exercise 77. Standing Hamstring Stretch 228
Exercise 78. Standing Quadriceps (Thigh) Stretch 230
Exercise 79. Standing Upper Back Stretch 231
Exercise 80. Standing Buttock and Back Stretch 233
Exercise 81. Standing Tricep and Lat Stretch 235
Exercise 82. Standing Chest and Shoulder Stretch 237
Exercise 83. Standing or Seated Neck Stretch 238

BREATHW**FOR YOUR BACK**RKS

Introduction

Do you look in the mirror and see slumped shoulders and a protruding abdomen?

Do you suffer from chronic low back pain or discomfort?

Have you been doing traditional abdominal exercises for years without any visible effect on your midsection?

Are you unable to do most exercises because back surgery or a back injury has lessened or restricted your movement?

Are you aware of tightness or tension in the neck or upper back much of the time?

Have you given up jogging or other aerobic exercise because it bothered your lower back?

Are you nagged by the feeling that the 125 crunches you do each time you go to the gym aren't doing you any good?

Do you want to look taller, leaner, shapelier, even younger?

If you answered "yes" to *any number* of these questions, then *this is the book for you.*

You are about to discover completely new ideas about exercise. You are beginning an adventure of self-awareness that will enhance your knowledge and understanding of how your body works. You will learn that slower, smaller, and more controlled movements are a safer and more effective way to strengthen your body. You will look slimmer, taller, and years younger by a simple change in your posture. You will discover that you can feel relaxed and invigorated after doing your exercises, rather than fatigued and sweaty, with an aching lower back.

You will learn a series of abdominal exercises that really work and, wonder of wonders, you have to do only a few of them at a time to achieve results. You can do them *wherever* you are, and you don't have to change clothes or even lie down on the floor. You can do them if you have a back injury, are recovering from an illness, are pregnant, or have just had a baby.

Cramping Your Style

The reason most people don't do abdominal exercises is pretty obvious. People don't do them because they are not enjoyable to do. In all my years of working with people and teaching exercise, I have not met anyone who *likes* doing abdominals. Not only are they not enjoyable, performing them can actually be *uncomfortable*. Curling up from a back lying position, over and over again, doesn't feel *good*. It strains your low back, hurts your neck, and just plain wears you out! I know men and women who religiously do the crunches and curl-ups at the end of their aerobics class and you can be sure that *none* of them likes to do crunches. I also know a lot of people who don't do any kind of abdominal strengthening. They have soft, thick midsections that are totally lacking in muscle tone. They get fatigued easily (particularly in their lower back region). They hate the way they look and they are always promising themselves to go on a diet and start doing crunches so they can "get rid of this belly."

So you're in for a treat. These abdominal exercises you're about to learn actually *feel* good and make *you* feel good. The unexpected reward for sticking with this program is that eventually you won't have to do the specific abdominal strengthening exercises every day. After a few months of doing them faithfully, your body will have integrated the basic movement into all your normal activities. Then you will be strengthening your abdominals all day long.

No Sweat

Our bodies are designed to enable us to use our arms in many
different positions during normal, functional movement. In
each different position the muscles in the chest, shoulders,
and back act as both prime movers and stabilizers of the arms,
shoulder girdle, and trunk. Changing the position of the arms
changes the function each muscle performs. Sometimes they
are lifting or pulling, sometimes they are pushing or turning,
sometimes they are slowing down the speed of the movement,
and sometimes they are holding bones in place. Performing a
variety of movements is what maintains balance in the muscle
groups. Since the Industrial Revolution most of our activity is
repetitive and involves moving the arms in only one or two
directions, over and over again. This limited, repetitive activity
contributes to muscle imbalances in the body and ultimately
affects the way the entire body moves.

In chapter 5, you will be introduced to range of motion
exercises that serve to loosen and warm the body up before
beginning the back strengthening program. They may also be
used as gentle strengthening exercises for those recovering
from an injury. They act as a stretch and a strengthener simultaneously and, when done regularly, will help you achieve improved range of motion and flexibility. These moves are done
slowly and fluidly, using the breath, and bring about a deep
state of relaxation. People have said that they are like doing
a moving meditation such as T'ai Chi, while lying on the floor.

Not only are these range of motion exercises pleasurable to
do, they allow the muscles to *practice* changing their function.
They restore *functional* balance within the muscles by encour-
aging the body to move synergistically, each muscle performing its specific function and other muscles assisting. As
you do these moves, you will be reinforcing your abdominal
strength by gently pulling in and up with your deep abdominal muscles.

I use the term "functional" often in this book. Functional
means that it applies to *practical* movement patterns of the
body. The movements you perform as you do your everyday
tasks, e.g., reaching, pulling, pushing, bending, stooping,
squatting, turning, etc.

The strengthening exercises for the back, in chapter 7, like the abdominal program, involve use of breathing techniques and very little movement. They are simple, straightforward, and very effective. They involve holding a contraction of the muscles in the back and shoulder girdle, with the arms, upper body, or legs held in a variety of positions that isolate each targeted muscle group.

Resistance is created by the gravitational pull against the body part being used as a lever. The angle and the distance of the arm or leg from the body is what determines which part of the muscle is being worked. These back strengthening exercises provide functional strength and they also establish good body mechanics. They each incorporate use of the deep abdominal muscles to provide stability for the trunk or middle of the body, and they all involve lengthening of the spine. By the way, good body mechanics simply means that you perform the movements efficiently and without undue stress to the body.

Lastly, you will learn a series of *moving* stretches in chapter 8 that will open you up, release the tension in your body, and make you *feel* wonderful.

The Ties That Bind

In the late 1940s and 1950, Herman Kabat, M.D., Ph.D., and two physical therapists, Margaret Knott and Dorothy Voss, conducted research that showed that the body moves primarily in spiral-diagonal patterns. Our muscles are attached to the bones at oblique or diagonal angles, and are sheathed and separated by connective tissue called *fascia*. This fascia is also layered throughout the body in diagonal directions.

Effective stretching should include and combine elements of this spiral-diagonal motion in order to assist the movement of the fascia over the muscles and to stretch the muscle attachments fully. The muscle attachments are where fibers at the end of the muscle continue into a strong, fibrous band, called a *tendon*, and attach to the bone.

The range of motion exercises and the moving stretches encourage a gradual increase in muscle length as you are doing the exercises by increasing the flow of blood and oxygen to the muscles and connective tissue. This lubricates the joints and decreases the tendency of the stretched muscles to return to their previously shortened position. The movements gently lengthen the fascia that binds the muscles together, and they help break up the collagen fibers of scar tissue that form to replace normal tissue when it's been injured.

Altered States

Because all the exercises and stretches are done with the eyes closed and use slow, deep breathing to enhance each move, they provide a total, effective release of muscular tension in the body as well as a profound sense of relaxation and well-being. If you do them daily, they will increase your overall strength and flexibility while you rejuvenate your body and calm your mind.

Here's something interesting for you: Simply sitting and resting or even going to sleep does not release the accumulated muscle tension that is created by stress. There are even some stages of sleep that initiate muscle tension and may cause us to thrash around in bed. Have you ever awakened in the morning curled into a tight fetal position or clutching your pillow and already feeling fatigued before you even get out of bed? The body needs to be told that it is safe to relax. It requires a conscious command; otherwise, it will stay in a perpetual state of readiness for fight or flight.

Throughout these exercises and stretches, you will focus your attention on your body. You will discover things about yourself you hadn't known. You will become aware of how your body collects and stores tension throughout the day. In my years of teaching exercise to a whole variety of age groups, sexes, and levels of physical conditioning, I've had one startling realization—most people are disconnected from their bodies! Even athletes in perfect condition don't always have the ability to *feel* what is happening in their bodies during normal movement or when they are exercising.

When I am working with private patients, they are always surprised to discover they were holding tension in a particular part of their body. They will be doing a move and assume they are keeping their body relaxed until I tell them to relax. Then their shoulders or hips will drop and they will realize they were actually tensing part of their body. No wonder they feel fatigued at the end of the day!

Promised Land

The 1990s have brought about a renaissance in fitness, health care, and exercise. Because we are now beginning to understand the connection between our bodies and our minds, the direction of our focus has changed. The approach to health has become more holistic. Many health care programs are now referred to as "wellness" programs. The ancient practices of holistic and homeopathic medicine have been resurrected, and healing through the touch of another person's hands is now accepted as credible treatment for illness. Chiropractic, massage, accupressure, and acupuncture are often covered by insurance companies, and meditation is accepted and used clinically for the relief of pain and the treatment of disease.

This book will introduce you to a philosophy and program of exercise that fits into this new direction of health care. The exercises will act as preventative and rehabilitative measures by restoring balance to the postural muscles and creating a strong internal corset of support. They will provide your body with renewed and increased energy as well as strength and flexibility. They address you as a *whole* person. They offer you the opportunity to get to know your body.

Going into the quiet place of intense concentration as you do the exercises allows you to *feel* sensations in your body that you haven't noticed before. This process quiets the internal chatter that fills your mind and often keeps you feeling fatigued and lacking in energy. Focusing your attention wholly on feeling your body as you do the exercises is like a meditation and is truly the practice of being in the moment.

A young man I had treated for back pain wrote me this letter:

I want to share the impact your exercises have had on my daily life. Before I worked with you I had no daily ritual in terms of abdominal or stretching exercises. Almost as soon as I tried the movements, I realized they were something I could weave into my day, to my benefit. As it happened at the time I was learning Qi-kung (Qi Gong). For the last four years each morning I have done a combination of the movements you taught me and the Taoist postures. It would be difficult to articulate how profound an effect this has had on my life. Not only are your exercises strengthening, calming, and a pleasure to perform, there is also a spiritual benefit. I have noticed that things that would once have knocked me off balance in my life no longer have that power. I believe the meditative quality of the exercises is as beneficial as the physical work itself. I plan on doing this for the rest of my life.

Connecting the Dots

I have written the book with different readers in mind. There is some clinical information about the anatomy of your body and then there is a lot of instruction that invites only your interpretation and imagination.

I am giving you the clinical information for a reason: you're entitled to an explanation of the function of a very precious possession—your body. You have a right to know how it works and why it may cause you pain. Pain is frightening. Pain is distracting. Pain interrupts and interferes with plans and activities. If you have been experiencing chronic pain or even mild discomfort for a long time, you may feel as though you no longer have control over your body's responses. This book can give that control back to you. Just knowing how the muscles work and how poor posture can contribute to back pain or headaches is a start. Understanding how improving your posture can alleviate some of the discomfort will motivate you to stay with this program and help you to manage your back pain. So don't be put off or frightened by some of the technical language. You have the ability to understand it, and I have made every effort to explain things in familiar terms.

In my twelve years of teaching exercise classes to many different types of individuals, I have found that people love to learn about their bodies. It gives them a sense of ownership. It instills a sense of pride and also of responsibility for taking care of that body. After all, your body is a gift, and it's the only one you've got.

School of Hard Knocks

In 1989 I owned a fitness center in Winter Park, Colorado. It wasn't just a business, it became my life. In addition to administrative duties I often found myself teaching more classes than was reasonable or even safe. I was fifty years old at the time and had been running every day for about fifteen years. I was never a competitive runner, but I did manage to run from three to five miles every morning. I was also lifting weights and doing hundreds of crunches in the course of teaching four or five classes every day. One day I began to experience pain in my lower back, and by the next morning I was in severe pain. I could hardly move. My injury was diagnosed as a bulging disc between the fourth and fifth lumbar vertebrae as a result of overuse and fatigue. The prescribed treatment was ice and rest, and I was advised that I should avoid bending forward from the waist. That advice wasn't hard to follow since I could not bend over or sit down without severe pain. Each time I drove my car it worsened my condition, and I even ate my meals standing up.

At the time, I believed, like most did, that crunches (small sit-ups) were the only way to strengthen the abdominal muscles. My injury presented a real problem: How could I teach abdominal strengthening exercises if I couldn't bend forward?

I frantically began to study my anatomy and physical therapy texts in search of answers. I learned that the *transversus abdominis* is the innermost layer of the abdominal wall. This muscle is referred to as the "corset muscle" because it acts like a girdle to pull in the abdomen. The transversus abdominis is attached to the diaphragm, which is the principal muscle of respiration. When you breathe in, the diaphragm contracts and pulls down, opening up the thoracic (chest) cavity. As this happens, the entire abdominal wall expands out. When you breathe out, it moves inward.

The physical therapy texts I read explained that forced expiration of breath caused a tightening of the entire abdominal wall. That gave me an idea. I began to experiment with breathing exercises. I found that by lying on my back and *actively pulling inward* as I exhaled, I could work the innermost layers of the abdominal wall. I could actually *feel* these muscles deep inside my body.

When doing the exercise with my knees bent, I tended to tense up and press down against the floor with my feet. I tried doing the same exercise passively, using a large roll or pillow under my knees. I immediately felt a lengthening of the abdominals when my legs were extended. By exhaling, pulling my abdominal muscles in, and holding them, I found I could go back to breathing and keep my tummy pulled in. But the exercise was still difficult to do without creating a lot of tension in the rest of my body.

I began taking a few minutes to relax before doing the exercise. I found that lying quietly with my eyes closed and visualizing the deep abdominal muscles slowed down my breathing and focused my attention on my body. Then when I did the forced expiration of breath and pulled the muscles in I could go back to breathing normally and the rest of my body stayed relaxed. My midsection began to change dramatically, and my abdominal strength increased. After a few weeks I no longer had to think about holding my stomach in. It appeared to be doing it on its own. More important, my back began to feel better!

Seeing Is Believing

I began to teach the exercise in my fitness center, and although my ideas originally met with resistance, I persisted and soon began to gain some support. Most of the members confided in me that their necks and backs had always felt strained after doing regular abdominal exercises. They acknowledged that these new exercises worked their abdominals without the neck and back discomfort. Soon people began to see the same changes in their posture and profile that I had.

Now, after many years of working with individuals suffering from chronic back pain and other conditions arising out of postural imbalances, the original exercises have developed into a complete program of strengthening, stabilizing, and stretching for the whole body. These "core" exercises focus on the deep muscles, strengthening the body from the inside out. This rehabilitative and preventive program also has the added advantage of changing the way the body looks.

Finally the most dramatic, unexpected benefit is your increased awareness of your body. You'll notice a distinct difference between how your body feels at rest and how you feel when you are moving. You will learn how to isolate and work a specific muscle or set of muscles, and how to relax isolated parts of your body. You will recognize muscle tension when it *begins* to develop, and know how to release it before it has time to accumulate and damage your body.

The combination of the exercises and self-awareness offers you an effective stress-relieving tool that you can take with you anywhere and use for the rest of your life. The result is an increased sense of inner balance and stability that is mirrored in the way you carry your body.

Here is how one of my clients describes the metamorphosis:

These exercises are like no other program I have done. They work! Their effectiveness can be felt while I am doing them because they work deep inside. The change has become a part of me rather than something temporary. Feeling the muscles each time I use them and getting visible results in a short time is very motivating. I've incorporated this program into my lifestyle and schedule easily, and that means that I'm still doing them!

So, get ready for an adventure. Be prepared to change your existing beliefs about exercise. You will need a large towel or pillow, comfortable clothes, and patience with yourself, since it takes time and practice to unlearn old habits and develop new ones.

Good work to you, and most of all, delight in this totally new experience!

1

Getting to the Core of the Matter

How would you like to get up in the morning and put on an undergarment that made you smaller all around, made you look taller and lighter, provided firm support for your lower back and your organs, and felt comfortable and flexible? In fact, what if you discovered you looked younger, felt better, and had more energy when you had it on? You would probably want to wear it every day, wouldn't you?

Currently, over 80 percent of the American population is suffering from some kind of back problem, primarily low back pain. A recent health newsletter from the Mayo Clinic (June 1996) stated that doctors treated seven million new cases of back pain in the last year. Insurance companies are spending over $16 billion each year on back injuries alone, and the average workman's compensation cost per employee, for this problem alone, is more than $7,000. It is no wonder many large companies require their employees to wear an elastic back support if they do any type of physical activity as part of their job. These wide elastic back supports resemble a kidney belt, and wrap around the body like a corset. The purpose of this corset is to provide external support for the lumbar spine.

Well, here's the good news. We have that same type of corset *inside* our own bodies! It is a highly underappreciated muscle called the transversus abdominis (Illustration 1), which performs exactly the same function as the elastic back support.

Illustration 1

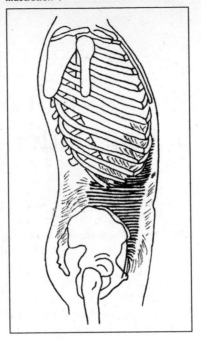

Transversus Abdominis

Layered over this muscle are the internal obliques (Illustration 2), which are composed of three sets of diagonal fibers that each perform slightly different functions. These two muscles—the transversus abdominis and the internal obliques—together make up what I call the deep internal girdle.

There are four muscles that make up the entire abdominal group. They are:

transversus abdominis
internal obliques
external obliques
rectus abdominis

Starting from *the inside out:* The transversus abdominis is the deepest layer of muscle. It draws in the abdominal wall

Illustration 2

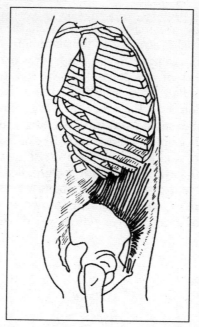

Internal Obliques

and works with the diaphragm to assist in respiration. The fibers of this muscle run horizontally (transversely), around the middle of the body, attaching on the bottom of the rib cage and around the top of the hips. As it contracts it compresses and supports the organs and contents of the abdomen in the body. When the transversus pulls inward, it lifts and supports the rib cage, actually lengthening the distance between the bottom of the ribs and the top of the hips. This is what creates the leaner and taller look. In doing this it acts as an important stabilizer of the trunk, by holding the rib cage and pelvis in correct relationship to one another. Weakness of this deep muscle results in a bulging out of the abdominal wall.

The internal obliques are the next layer of muscle. Because the fibers run in diagonal directions, they duplicate the action of the original Platex girdle by creating a second panel of support. They also help hold your guts in the pelvic cavity, and aid in respiration by working together with the transversus abdominis. They are major stabilizers of the trunk, and are the primary muscle responsible for alignment of the pelvis. As the lower fibers contract in a slightly upward direction, they rotate the *bottom* of the pelvis forward, creating a pelvic tilt. This results in a flatter lower abdomen as well as correct alignment of the pelvis to the rib cage. They are involved at a deep level, in flexion and rotation (twisting), from side to side.

The external obliques (Illustration 3) are a more superficial layer of muscle, and although they *assist* in stabilization and respiration, their primary function is trunk flexion and rotation. These are the muscles you use whenever you turn to look over your shoulder, when you reach down to the side to pick up a suitcase or briefcase, or when you do any type of curl-

Illustration 3

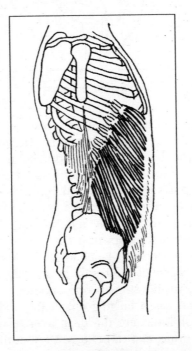

External Obliques

up or crunch with a twisting motion. Although like the internal obliques, their muscle fibers are diagonal, they are attached more to the front of the body and do not have the ability to pull the abdomen in like the deeper muscles do.

Last, the most superficial muscle—the one closest to the outside of the body—is the rectus abdominis (Illustration 4). It is the primary muscle used when doing any type of sit-up, curl-up, or crunch. The muscle fibers run vertically down the front of the body, from the fifth, sixth, and seventh ribs to the crest of the pubic symphysis or pubic bone. It resembles a pair of flank steaks because of the tendon insertion separating the two halves. It has six other tendonous attachments that run across the muscle horizontally, forming the famous "six pack." This muscle basically has one function: flexion. It brings the rib cage and pelvis closer together by either flexing the trunk forward or curling the pelvis upward. It cannot compress the abdomen. In other words, *its function has nothing to do with holding the stomach in.*

Illustration 4

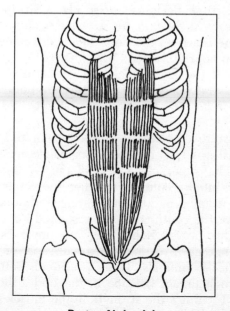

Rectus Abdominis

Traditional abdominal exercises have focused on the rectus abdominis and the external obliques to achieve the ever-elusive flat tummy and to strengthen the abdominals as support for the lower back. The problem with that logic is that these are the two most superficial layers of muscle in the abdominal group. As I've just explained, holding in your abdomen is not the primary function of these muscles. Flexion and rotation are, and they can only *assist* in stabilization. Only the deep layers of muscle—the transversus abdominis and the internal obliques—serve that function. They create a solid center from which to build out. That's why I called these exercises that develop these deep layers core exercises.

All of the abdominal muscles are bound together, connected by layers of connective tissue, and insert into a broad tendon called the *linea alba,* which runs down the center of the abdomen. When you work the deep muscles by pulling them in, you automatically strengthen the more superficial layers of muscle.

Unfortunately, it does not work the other way around. Any type of front trunk flexion exercise like a sit-up, curl-up, or crunch, causes a slight *bulging out* of the abdominal wall as you lift up. Lie down on the floor, bend your knees, and place your hands on your abdomen. Now lift your head. You should be able to feel the abdominal wall get hard and push out. This action is the opposite of pulling the abdominal wall in, and a firmly *pulled in* abdomen is what provides support for your back.

I ran a test to compare the exercises in this program to traditional curl-ups and crunches using electromagnetic testing equipment. The superficial layers of muscle actually experienced a more intense contraction when the subject performed the exercises in my program than during traditional abdominal exercises. Plus, the contraction was sustained for a longer time. What does this prove? Something you never thought you'd hear. You don't have to do sit-ups, curl-ups, or crunches to strengthen the abdominals. There is a much better way!

In order to maintain balance in the body, there needs to be a ratio of 1½ times the strength in the muscles that extend the body (pull the body backward) vs. the muscles that flex the body (bend the body forward). Overworking the rectus abdominis doing flexion exercises like crunches creates excessive tightness of that muscle and results in a shortening or pulling down of the body. It depresses the rib cage as well as compressing the abdominal contents. It limits the ability to breathe fully and affects both digestion and elimination.

The exercises in this program strengthen the deepest layers of abdominal muscle *and* and rectus abdominis.

The Naked Truth

The bony structures of the body are designed to support and carry our weight. The muscles were designed to hold our bony parts together in correct relationship to one another and to pull our bones together, which produces movement. Our muscles were not meant to support weight.

Standing involves synergistic coordination of bones, ligaments, tendons, muscles, and fascia, so that the body is stable as a whole. Our skeletons are supported over our feet by passive tension of the ligaments, by the elastic property of our muscles, and by connective tissue called *fascia* that holds it all together. In relaxed standing there is only a minimal amount of activity in the muscles that act as a stabilizing force. These antigravity muscles produce small amounts of activity that maintain the body in an upright position by a very slight constant swaying. This is believed to be an automatic neurological reflex to relieve stress on the joints.

Good posture protects the supporting structures of our body against undue stress or injury in all the positions you can assume—e.g., standing, sitting, squatting, stooping, and so forth. With good posture your muscles can function efficiently and optimally. Poor posture, on the other hand, creates stress and strain on all the systems of the body and will eventually affect your normal function. (More about this in later chapters.)

Let's talk about some of the negative things that can occur in your back and neck when your abdominal muscles are overstretched and weakened.

When the abdominal wall protrudes there is an increased

gravitational pull forward and down on the body, allowing the abdominal contents to bulge out of the pelvic cavity. The front (anterior) muscles in the chest wall are then pulled into a shortened position, which creates an increased pull on the muscles in the upper back. They become overstretched. The result is a rounded posture (Illustration 5). In order to keep the eyes horizontal and level, the body will adapt by moving the head forward and tilting it back, thereby creating shortened, tight muscles in the back of the neck.

Your head moving away from the axis, or center line, of your body creates further negative impact. Every inch it moves forward it increases the compression force in the back of your

Illustration 5

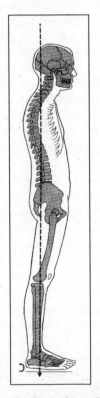

Rounded Posture (Sway-Backed)

neck (lower cervical spine) by adding its own weight. Your head is normally one-tenth of your body weight. An average human head weighs between 12 and 20 pounds. If an adjustment in your posture moves it 1 inch off center, it can produce the compressive load of a 25- to 40-pound head.

When the muscles in your neck and upper back are held in an imbalanced position, your shoulders tend to rotate forward. With your chest dropped and your midsection shortened, the muscles that are involved in diaphragmatic breathing are compromised and the breathing muscles that assist them are overworked.

What results is an aged, hunched-over, closed-in posture—a posture that looks less energetic, less fit than one that is lengthened and well balanced. When you look in the mirror, what do *you* see?

Take a look at the pictures of different postures (Illustration 6). These are fairly classic and also exaggerated or extreme cases, but you may identify with one of them. Go stand in front of a mirror (full length, if possible) in your underwear. Now, look at yourself from the front. What do you see? Do your shoulders look droopy, your chest caved in, and your belly protruding? Do you look as if you collapsed into your pelvis, or do you see a lifted chest and open, relaxed shoulder area? Can you see a hint of a waistline because your abdomen is being supported by muscles? Are your legs fairly straight, or are your feet either turned too far out or too far in?

Now turn to the side. Use a hand mirror and take a good look at your posture. Which picture do you resemble the most? The one with the most exaggerated low back curve and bulging abdominal wall or the flat back or swayback postures? Look at the ideal posture (Illustration 7). See where the plumb line is. See how the body is balanced? Now what about you? Take your time and honestly evaluate what you see. Does your body look well supported? Does it look balanced and energetic? Look at your upper back. Is the curve within normal ranges or is it overly rounded so that your chest is dropped and hollow? Where is the position of your head in relation to the rest of your body? Is it centered? Are your knees locked (hyperextended), or are they bent even when you are standing

Illustration 6

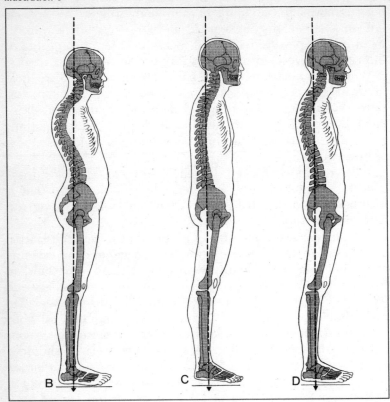

Various Postures

up straight because your hamstrings are so tight? Notice where your pelvis is. Is it fairly well aligned under your rib cage or is it tilted too far backward or forward?

If you look like the picture of ideal posture, congratulations! You won't have to improve your posture, but you now have a tool to *maintain* that good posture and abdominal tone for the rest of your life. But if you're not happy with what you see, don't despair. You can improve your posture or anything else. That's what this program is all about—bringing *your* body back into balance.

Illustration 7

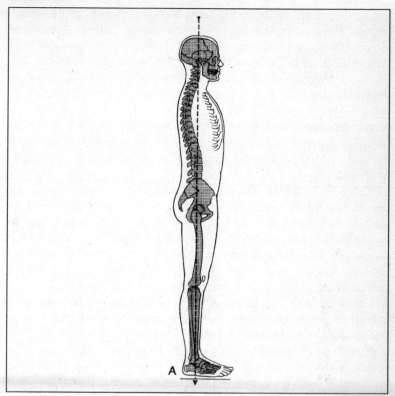

A

Ideal Posture

Stacking It Up

The lower back (lumbar spine), can respond to the pressures
I've just described by either increasing its curve or lessening
it. Either one of these responses creates a set of adaptations
by other muscles in the pelvis, buttocks, and legs that can
cause further stresses on your body. These directly affect the
muscles in your back, hip flexors, gluteals (buttocks), and hamstrings. The muscles on the inside and outside of your thighs
are also affected. All play a major role in low back pain. We
will talk more about that in chapters 5 and 6.

John McM. Mennell, M.D., one of the foremost experts on the musculoskeletal system, introduced the world to the concept of the mechanical body as a complete system of its own. He established that a normally functioning musculoskeletal system is essential to health in all the other systems.

The musculoskeletal system is very much like a stack of dominos. If one of the dominos is out of alignment, the entire stack is precariously balanced. This is the theory known as serial distortion, which states that from an area of weakness or misalignment, weakness and imbalance will radiate both up and down the skeletal frame. The entire body's alignment is affected.

There is a lot of discussion and even controversy about which part of the body is most important in terms of alignment. The question is, Which part of the body is the one to create the dysfunctional response in the rest of the body? One school of thought believes the head is the pivotal point of balance and alignment for the body. Another group believes the position of the pelvis establishes our balance.

I believe both the pelvis and head alignment are of equal importance, and therefore focus my attention on the area central to both of those locations: *the abdomen.* For our purposes, it doesn't really matter which created the initial problem. The result is that the whole body is adversely affected. Focusing on what I call the core establishes a place of stability and strength in the center. The results I've seen have been exclusively positive.

Let's go back to elastic back supports for a moment. One of the problems with them is that the people who wear them, either as a preventive measure or as part of their rehabilitation following a back injury, have a greater percentage of new or recurring injuries after they remove the corset. Because it is external, it removes the need for the body's own musculature to do even minimal stabilization. They actually serve to *weaken* stabilizing muscles. The message the body gets is *Don't bother to protect yourself, the corset will do it for you.*

The back was designed with three gentle but necessary curves, a forward curve in the neck (cervical region), a backward curve in the upper back (thoracic region), and a forward curve in the low back (lumbar region). The curves in the neck and lower back are created by the wedge-shaped intervertebral discs and cause the spine to curve around the invisible plumb line that runs through the center of the body. This provides a better means of balancing and distributing the weight of the body on the vertebral column. The discs not only act as cushions and shock absorbers, they also allow slight movement between the vertebrae.

Each disc is made up of two parts—an outer plate of cartilage-like material, and a soft center. The center consists of collagen fibers in a gelatinlike protein material that is 70 to 85 percent water. This softness allows it to change shape and accounts for the ability of the disc to withstand compression. Pressure upon the discs results in dehydration. Each day, our weight-bearing activities press minute quantities of water out of the discs and into the bloodstream. As the discs lose their water content, they become thinner, and this can result in a loss of height of up to as much as ¾ inch in a mature adult in a single day. When pressure on the discs is relieved, as it is when you're in bed at night, water is reabsorbed from the bloodstream, and the discs expand to their former size.

From the age of thirty on, a slow process of disc degeneration takes place caused mainly by a decrease in the water content in the soft center of the disc. In young adults the disc contains about 85 percent water. With aging, this percentage drops dramatically as the ability of the disc to reabsorb water decreases. As a result, the disc becomes thinner and weaker. These weakened discs become increasingly vulnerable, and under excessive pressure or strain they can bulge or rupture.

Measurements of pressure in the lumbar spine have shown that there is between 200 to 300 pounds of compressive force on a single disc when you're standing. If you hold 20 additional pounds of weight in your hands, the pressure on the disc increases by over 200 pounds, especially if you lean forward. The more you lean forward, the more the pressure is increased.

Although the vertebral column is flexible and can bend and rotate in many directions, it also serves a protective function. It encases the delicate spinal cord and the spinal nerves, which exit through a small opening in each vertebra. When a disc bulges, or herniates, it pushes out from between the vertebrae and can put pressure on the nerve root. This can result in pain, either mild or acute, tingling and numbness in the legs, and even loss of strength and muscle function. This is where the function of our *internal corset* comes into play.

As you inhale, the diaphragm pulls down and this puts pressure against the inner wall of the transversus. When you are doing the basic In and Up move, this push creates resistance as the muscle fibers of the transversus abdominis hold against the pressure. This is called *intra-Abdominal* pressure. Studies have indicated that this intraabdominal pressure can reduce the compression in the lumbar spine by 50 percent. That is a significant improvement over the external back support that is reported to reduce compression by only 30 percent and actually *causes* more problems than it cures!

Another wonderful thing about this internal corset is that it lines up the dominos. It "stacks" the body in correct (or closer to correct) alignment.

The reason I add "closer to correct" alignment is that even though pulling in the deepest layer of the abdominal wall automatically stabilizes the rib cage and lengthens the spine, you can't force the body from poor posture into good posture. You need to relax and lengthen the shortened, tight muscles that held the body in the poor posture.

That's why this program includes *conscious* belly breathing, range of motion exercises, and a whole series of *moving* stretches that loosen the body up, establish new muscle memory patterns, and allow you to relax and get to know and care for your body.

It's the Principle of the Matter

The exercises that follow focus on the two deepest layers of abdominal muscles, the transversus abdominis and the internal obliques. The two more superficial muscles are also strengthened during these exercises, but by using your breath and focusing on the deepest muscles, the tightening begins from the inside out.

This is how it works. When you inhale, the diaphragm contracts and pulls down into the body, thereby opening up the chest cavity to receive two hearty lungs full of air. When this happens, the transversus abdominis expands, allowing movement of the abdominal organs out of the way, so that the lungs can fill. Once the lungs have filled with air, the diaphragm releases its contraction and pushes the air out of the lungs with some force. The transversus abdominis assists in this action by contracting inward and squeezing the diaphragm upward. This is a highly simplified but accurate description of what happens. Since the transversus abdominis *has* to expand when you inhale and *contract* when you exhale, the muscle fibers experience resistance or *stress* if you hold them in while you breathe normally. This kind of stress is what causes the muscle fibers to increase their strength in order to function to their maximum capacity. In other words, *breathing* while you hold your abdominals in and up will make them stronger.

You will also be using your muscles in one of their primary functions: stabilization. The abdominal exercises use the pulling in and tightening of your muscles to put the rib cage and pelvis in correct alignment, thereby stabilizing your lumbar spine. You add resistance to these muscles by moving various parts of your body. Because muscles that are attached to the rib cage are also attached to the arm and shoulder girdle, movement of the arms creates a pull and change of position in the upper body. The latissimus dorsi muscles in the back originate from the top of the hip bones, cross over the bottom of the scapula, and attach on the inside of the upper arm. In this case, movement of the arms puts a pull on the pelvis. All this movement adds considerable resistance to the abdominal muscles, as they work to hold the rib cage and pelvis in correct alignment with each other and stabilize your back.

Movement of your arms upward toward your head normally involves stabilization by your back muscles. In the exercises that involve motion, you are not only working the muscles in your back functionally, but as you are keeping tension in your abdominals you create an *eccentric* contraction because the abdominals are being lengthened against resistance.

The same principle applies to the exercises that involve

movement of your legs. Although your abdominal muscles do
not directly raise or move your legs, they are affected by the
muscles in your upper thigh (both front and back) that are
attached to your pelvis. Movement of your legs alters the position of your pelvis, and any change in position of either your
rib cage or your pelvis affects both your abdominals and
your back.

Now, look at the pictures of the abdominal muscles again.
Notice the direction of the muscle fibers. As you pull your
abdomen in, the transversus abdominis, the internal obliques,
and the external obliques contract and rotate your pelvis.
When you are lying on your back this action will curl your
pubic bone up toward your chest like a scorpion's tail, to
flatten your lower back against the floor. (This is the reason for
the *in and up* instructions during the exercises.) The muscles
maintain your rib cage and pelvis in correct alignment with
each other during movement of your arms and legs. Maintaining stability of your rib cage and back during the exercises
is the way your abdominal muscles are strengthened.

When a muscle contracts, the fibers *slide* into each other.
They compress in much the same way you collapse a telescope
or a radio antenna. This is called a *concentric contraction*. A
muscle may shorten up to 50 percent of its normal length
when maximally contracted. As a muscle contracts, the tension
actually *decreases* because the workload is being shared by a
greater number of muscle fibers. When a muscle is *lengthened*
while it is still holding a contraction, there is a lot of stress
on the individual fibers because as it pulls apart there are
fewer fibers holding the tension. This is called an *eccentric
contraction*. You can replicate the action by interlacing your
fingers, tightening the muscles in your hand, and then trying
to pull your fingers apart. See what I mean? All the latest
research indicates that eccentric contractions are what create
the most effective work for the muscles.

Keeping your muscles "pulled in" while you are using them
as stabilizers and "pulled in" while you are continuing to
breathe diaphragmatically is the ultimate strengthener for
these deep abdominals.

As your muscles get stronger and tighter, the "pulled-in"

look becomes something you can maintain, even during normal, everyday activity. Thinking "in and up" becomes part of your consciousness and *pulling* in the abdominals when you exhale becomes the way you breathe. Soon you are working your abdominals all day long.

The Breath of Life

There has been a lot written recently about the importance of our breath to our total health and well-being. From all the attention, you'd think someone had just discovered it! Eastern cultures have been practicing conscious breathing for thousands of years. The martial arts all involve conscious use of the breath, as well as the meditative movements such as T'ai Chi and Chi-Kung. All forms of Yoga use the breath as the central component to establish concentration, rhythm, and strength. Relaxation training and meditation used to control pain are also based on slow, deep breathing.

The body needs only six to nine breaths a minute. The hectic nature of our lives, with our crammed schedules, crowded freeways, and constantly ringing telephones, keeps us from breathing as slowly and fully as we should. As we become stressed we unconsciously begin to take shorter, shallower breaths. The average person takes between ten to twenty-one breaths each minute. The faster our rate of respiration, the more anxious we feel. Soon we are operating in the fight or flight mode, and the entire body is affected. Because the brain requires three times more oxygen than the rest of the body, our concentration is affected. We feel scattered and distracted.

As we get older, our muscle tissue changes. It loses its elasticity and becomes restricted. Unless we actively do something to counteract it, the normal aging process reduces the amount of air we breathe by restricting the ability of the rib cage to expand. If we don't improve our breathing habits, we can decrease our breathing capacity by thirty to forty gallons of air an hour by the time we are in our seventies.

Slow belly breathing stimulates the parasympathetic nervous system, which allows your muscles to relax and removes their need for additional oxygen. This enables you to breathe easily throughout the execution of the exercises. Belly breathing or diaphragmatic breathing has significant positive effect on the function of the heart. It decreases heart rate, it reduces systolic blood pressure, it reduces the sympathetic nervous system response, and it affects the ebb and flow of a process called *respiratory sinus arrhythmia*. Respiratory sinus arrhythmia refers to the way the heart responds during respiration. The heart rate speeds up when you inhale, and it slows down as you exhale. This ebb and flow of the breath, which creates a rising and falling pressure, massages the vascular walls. The pulsating pressure flushes the walls of the arteries and helps them remain smooth and supple.

Belly breathing also *actively* stretches the entire abdominal wall and is therefore an important component in recreating and maintaining elasticity in the muscle fibers. The effects of actively stretching a muscle are very different from what happens when you allow a muscle to remain in an overstretched position. When they remain in an overstretched position, the muscles become weakened and permanently overstretched. By slowing down your inhalation and exhalation as you belly breathe, you assist your muscles in their expansion and contraction response, and this enhances the elasticity in the muscle fibers.

Feeling Your Way Around

Exercise physiologists have been investigating the mind-body connection for years. It appears that when the attention is focused on a particular area of the body or muscle group, the response from those muscles is stronger. The theory is that concentration intensifies the message to the muscle fibers to either contract or relax.

Paying attention to what you are feeling as you belly breathe allows your active participation in the stretching and lengthening of the muscles and connective tissue in the front of the chest and shoulder area. You will establish new memory patterns in your back muscles as you consciously relax and let go of tension in your back while maintaining an improved postural position.

This feeling is *proprioception*. Proprioception (pro-pree-o-sep-shun) is the *awareness* of stimulation in the tissues of the body by nerve endings. Pain is a proprioceptive sensation. So is itching or tingling or that tightness you sometimes feel in your neck or between your shoulder blades. Noticing where your weight is on your feet when you are standing is also proprioception. In other words, it is being aware of how your body moves (or is quiet) in space.

By alternating your focus of attention from the muscles being strengthened to the muscles you want to stay relaxed, you will develop the skill of *proprioceptive isolation*. This increased awareness is a necessary and valuable tool in the release of the tension you accumulate in your body every day.

Many of the strengthening exercises and stretches involve holding a position for several seconds to strengthen the muscles. Slowly releasing the tension in the muscles being strengthened and in the muscles being stretched assists in the development of new memory patterns in the tissues. Your muscles are inherently elastic and when released quickly after being stretched or shortened will return to their normal resting length. As I said earlier, they don't have the ability to lengthen, but they do return to their normal position. So if your chest area is tighter than your upper back, or your hamstrings are tighter than the front of your thighs, that's what your body will try to return to. By letting the tension slowly dissolve without altering your body position (I call it "sneaking out" of the contraction), you reduce the recoil response that normally follows.

If you do the exercises and stretches daily, at the end of thirty days or sooner you will see a dramatic difference in your midsection and your posture.

The Long and the Short of It

The abdominal exercises begin with the easiest ones and progress to the difficult ones, as you work against greater and greater resistance. There are a lot of exercises, but don't be overwhelmed by their number. *It is absolutely not necessary to do the entire program to achieve results.* I created many different exercises to offer variety and because not every exercise is for everyone. Each exercise has a different component of resistance, depending upon the position of the arms or the legs. Some involve movement of a body part, some do not. If, owing to age, injury, pregnancy, or any other condition, including lack of time, you are only able to do the first three exercises, you will see results. If you only enjoy or feel comfortable doing one or two of *any* of the exercises, you will feel results, and you can increase the intensity of those exercises to speed up your progress.

It is important to read through each exercise before you do it. The instructions are detailed and easy to follow. There is information about ordering audio cassettes of the exercises at the back of the book.

The program is completely flexible. If you have no disability or restrictions to keep you from doing the whole program, then you have a wonderful tool that can be changed and adjusted to fit your strength and fit into your schedule. You can pick out two or three of your favorites and just do those every day or you can try a new one every day. Do whichever exercises are easiest and most comfortable. This is a completely unstructured program. There are no have tos.

Remember that eventually your body will be doing the basic move on its own. The program you're about to learn is more accurately described as neuromuscular reeducation then an exercise program requiring strict adherence to form. First you learn the concept, then you learn how to do the physical pulling in of the abdominal wall. You'll get stronger by gradually increasing resistance and being consistent in performing a few exercises every day. Soon you'll incorporate them into your everyday activities. The power of this program is its simplicity.

All in a Day's Work

As I said earlier, it is not necessary to do the whole abdominal program every day. In its entirety it would take from thirty to forty-five minutes. If you only have five or ten minutes a day, then choose just two of any of the abdominal exercises. You can do them together or at different times during the day.

For instance, you could do the floor or bed-lying exercises the minute you wake up in the morning or the last thing at night before retiring. If you sleep on a firm mattress, the basic Supine In and Up and side-lying exercises can even be done while you are still in bed. Just pull your pillow out from under your head, stick it under your knees, and go to it. How easy can it get?

Both the Forced Expiration of Breath and the Wall Standing are perfect for short work breaks throughout the day. Get up from your desk for a few minutes and go find a wall or go into the rest room at work and stand in front of the mirror. These two exercises are wonderful stress management tools, so use them every chance you get. The weight-bearing exercises are the ones that will functionally reinforce the move the fastest.

When you are at home doing housework, get down on the floor and do the In and Up on Hands and Knees. You can lean over your kitchen counter at home or your desk at work for a modified version of the In and Up. No one even needs to know you are doing these exercises. Do the In and Up move in your car while you are sitting in traffic (might as well put that time to use!), or do the sitting exercise at your desk.

People I have worked with find a variety of ways to integrate the exercises into their busy schedules. Many say they do the In and Up move while driving. One woman does them in the middle of the night if she wakes up and can't go back to sleep. Another does them whenever she is standing in her kitchen cooking or doing dishes. Several women have told me they pull In and Up while standing in line at the grocery store.

A physician at the hospital where I teach wrote me a note about the difference the program made in his life:

They (the exercises) taught me how to "carry" my body in a way that made sense immediately but was not among the common wisdoms. Now I can stand at the operating table for extended periods of time without the usual fatigue and pain.

A sixty-year-old female client who had had multiple surgeries felt a dramatic difference after several months on my program:

> When I began your exercises I was still having problems with low back pain and spasms, and limited range of motion and tenseness in neck and shoulders. I had been using a pillow under my knees and a roll under my waist at night all these years. It has been three months since I no longer needed the pillow or roll to be comfortable. The leg cramps, random muscle twitching, and spasms in my left leg I once experienced nightly are now infrequent. I have almost full range of motion in my neck and arms. The focus on sensing specific muscle action has helped me to exercise more effectively, resulting in better muscle tone and posture.

All my clients tell me they stand up straighter and now catch themselves slouching—things they had never paid attention to before. The letter I received from the woman who created Woman's Way Ski Seminars says it all:

> Of all the pleasures and benefits that the exercises have given me, the most exciting thing is seeing the changes in my body, my bearing, and movement. When I unexpectedly glimpse my reflection in a mirror, or see an unposed snapshot of myself, I say a word of thanks for the positive changes that the exercises brought into my life.

For those who work at a computer (almost everyone these days), I suggest setting a timer on your computer to remind you to take a break and do Forced Expiration or Wall Standing at least twice during the workday. You can use the marquee screen saver program to scroll In and Up on your monitor as a reminder to pull your abdominals in and breathe correctly. See how quickly it becomes ingrained into your consciousness.

Sound crazy? Try it. These simple exercises are designed to fit into your daily life with minimal fuss. You don't need special clothes, special equipment, or big blocks of time. You won't get sweaty, so you can do them at work and go on with your day. You can take five minutes here and there and do much of the program every day.

Sticking to Your Guns

Being consistent is important. You are choosing to do two things: let go of old habits and beliefs about exercise, and create new ones. In order to create a new habit, you need to be ritualistic in your devotion for about twenty-one days. Suddenly, what required conscious effort begins to feel natural.

If you do the abdominals every day, you will be able to *feel* the difference within three or four days, and *see* a difference in your midsection at the end of two to three weeks. It will be slight, but you should see the hint of an indentation on each side of your abdomen underneath the ribs. At the end of those first few weeks you should also notice an improvement in the way your back feels, and you'll feel stronger.

At the end of a month you should be able to see a change in your abdominals. You will be able to hold your stomach in with less effort, and you will notice a pulled-in look under your ribs. At the end of two months of daily abdominals, people will comment on how much leaner you look, and your energy level and confidence about your looks will have improved dramatically.

I love these next two letters. They show just how diverse your experience can be with these exercises. You will benefit from them, whether you have back pain or not!

What I discovered about your abdominal exercises is most profound when I don't do them! As a middle-aged woman, my abdominal area tends to "pouch" and round in unflattering ways. When I do your exercises, it is amazing how much flatter my stomach is, how much sleeker my body looks, and how much younger I appear. My body seems "long and lean" because my posture is tremendously improved. If I didn't do your exercises I would look like a typical middle-aged woman who didn't take care of her body.

Originally I took your class because I wanted to look good wearing a form-fitting evening gown to a ball. Four weeks later, I did wear the gown, looked great, and told everyone that it was the result of doing your amazing abdominal exercises. Thank you for teaching me a spectacular way to look great. The exercises are easy to understand, feel good to do and are very relaxing.

The following letter came from a fifty-year-old woman who was referred to me by a chiropractor. She had scoliosis and had suffered from severe back pain for many years. She improved tremendously as a result of doing the exercises consistently.

I was so impressed and delighted with the exercises you taught me. I was amazed to see and feel the results I achieved in only two weeks of doing them twice a day, and will continue them forever. My lower back continues to improve, and I believe that strengthening that "girdle" around the spinal column was what did it. The relaxation I feel from the deep belly breathing is wonderful. I feel I have an extra and important bonus.

Getting *Back* to Health

You need to do the back-strengthening exercises only two or three times a week to feel marked improvement. The back exercises followed by one or two of the moving stretches will take about thirty minutes. To achieve results, you must do all the back exercises. Although I suggest you do them after warming up with the range of motion moves, they can be done separately if your time is limited. Again, it's the consistency with which you do the exercises that will increase the strength of your muscles and bring about desired changes in your posture.

As with the abdominal exercises, the back exercises are as much about reeducating your muscles as they are about strengthening them. Because each exercise is a sustained, exaggerated version of positions we strike in everyday movement, your body will become *functionally* strong. The good news is that there will come a time when you will no longer need to do the structured exercise program every day. If you're consistent in the beginning, your posture will change and your body will begin supporting itself. Your muscles will stay strong and balanced because you are *using* them to hold your body in your improved posture. Once you've achieved that functional strength—and you will—you can cut back to a shorter routine.

Choose just one or two of the exercises that reinforce your new posture and allow your body to move differently from what you do in your everyday activities. Do those exercises once or twice a week as a reminder to your muscles. This will keep you from returning to your former posture. If you catch yourself starting to slouch again, go back on the entire program for a couple of weeks.

You will want to approach the range of motion exercises and stretches differently. Both require more of your time, but they are so relaxing that my clients think of them as something they can't wait to do rather than something they have to do.

If you try to rush through them in a hurry, you are likely to create more tension than you release. You won't enjoy the experience either. If you choose a time when you can relax, you will *feel* the delicious sensation of your body gradually letting go of its tension as you surrender into each position. You will *feel* your range of motion expanding as you do the stretches, and after working through them a few times, you will begin to see a permanent increase in your range of motion that will last from one stretch session to another.

It helps if you can pick a time when you are least likely to be interrupted by the phone or other people. Playing soothing music may also help you to relax. I suggest and hope that you make time for these moves every day. But if it is difficult for you to find the time to do them every day (the whole sequence takes about thirty minutes), you will still achieve results if you do them every other day. You can alternate between the range of motion moves one day and the stretches the next. Chances are you probably don't devote much time to getting to know your body or listening to the messages it is sending you. These stretches are a wonderful way to start the day, to end it, or both! The entire program—two or three abdominals, the range of motion moves, the back-strengthening exercises, and the stretches—takes approximately an hour.

When you begin the program your focus should be on strengthening the deep abdominals and relaxing and lengthening the shortened muscles in the chest, shoulders, and lower back. For the first two weeks, do the abdominal exercises, the range of motion exercises, and the moving stretches. After that, the strengthening of the other weak muscles should begin. Working the muscles in this manner develops increased strength and stability at the core level and results in improved posture, reduced back problems and discomfort, better respiratory function, and dramatically improved abdominal tone. Remember, we are strengthening from the inside out.

Don't hesitate to look for conclusive evidence that the exercises are working. Before you start the program, measure your waist and abdomen, standing in your normal, relaxed posture. Write down the measurements. At the end of the first and second month, measure again, using your new relaxed posture. Notice the difference!

The exercises are grouped together by chapter. You are guided through each exercise as though you were with a personal instructor (that's why they're so long!), so *read each exercise through before attempting it.* You will learn how many repetitions to do and how to combine the exercises to make them more effective and efficient. The illustrations of the exercises will show you the proper position and direction of each movement.

Don't be discouraged if you can't remember the exercises exactly; the principle of pulling in is what's important. If you don't do the exercises precisely the way I describe them, it's no big deal. If you purchase the audio cassette of the exercises, it will allow you to completely relax. (See page 249 for more info.) You can also record your own voice reading the exercise instructions.

Seniors, pregnant women, handicapped individuals, or those recovering from an injury or surgery should look at the end of each exercise under Special Tips. I've included modifications that will allow almost everyone to do the exercises safely and comfortably. So . . .

GET YOUR TOWEL AND LET'S GET STARTED!

PART I

Abdominal Strengthening Program

2

Basic Training
(Or Exercise That Doesn't
Feel Like Exercise)

Belly Breathing, the Miracle Worker

Most people breathe in reverse. We don't start out that way, but the older we get, the more we restrict, tighten, and shorten our body movements. Breathing in reverse is just one of the ways we do that. What is breathing in reverse? If I asked you to stand or sit up straight and breathe deeply, what would you do? Most people expand the chest first and draw in the abdomen. As they exhale, they let their chests fall and the muscles in the abdomen relax and drop. They have a forward slouch on the exhale rather than a lifting and opening up of the chest.

This is how healthy breathing works: On inhalation, the abdomen expands, the rib cage lifts and expands, and the diaphragm contracts, drawing the air in and filling our lungs. The oxygen, which is 21 percent of the air we breathe, enters little chambers in the lungs and then passes through the membranes of the lungs directly into the red blood cells in our bloodstream. The hemoglobin within the cell carries the oxygen to all the cells in our body, which is what keeps us alive. Now gravity pulls most of the blood supply into the lower portion of the lungs, so the air needs to be drawn all the way down into the lungs to oxygenate the blood.

Reverse breathing, which is chest breathing, doesn't allow

the abdominal muscles to expand or allow complete ventilation of the lungs. The oxygen-rich air that we breathe only fills the upper portion of the lungs. It never reaches the lower lungs or the bloodstream. The result is a 25 percent decrease in oxygen in our bloodstream as we get older. This affects the heart, the skeletal muscles, and all the organs, including the brain. It affects *all* the tissues in the body. Over time, the lungs lose their elasticity and can no longer expand fully.

A young, healthy adult breathes in approximately 135 gallons of air every hour. Reverse breathing cuts that capacity down to about 95 gallons an hour. The difference is as much as it would take to walk 2 miles.

When you're belly breathing, you allow your abdomen (as well as your chest) to fully expand outward when you inhale and to move in as you exhale. Belly breathing actively involves all the muscles of respiration and brings life-sustaining oxygen to all the other muscles in the body.

By combining belly breathing with forced expiration of breath, you turn a normal function into a strengthening move.

Belly breathing plays an important role in the following exercises. First of all, it stretches the muscles in the abdomen *actively,* as opposed to allowing the muscles to become overstretched (and therefore weakened) from lack of use. Whenever you are working to strengthen a muscle, both lengthening and shortening moves are necessary to create and maintain elasticity in the fibers. Belly breathing does just that. If you consciously breathe through your nose, belly breathing helps the body to achieve a state of complete relaxation. During the relaxation response our need for oxygen is decreased. The heart rate drops and breathing becomes slow and shallow. This slowing process makes it easier to hold your abdominals in tightly and still breathe comfortably. Lastly, active belly breathing reinforces the message your abdominals have probably forgotten: that they were designed to move outward on inhalation, pull inward during exhalation.

I received the following letter from one of the students in my classes, who happens to be an elite senior athlete. Although in her sixties, she races cross country and skate-skis, and is also a serious kayaker:

The development of a strong girdle of support has enabled me to lengthen my spine by lifting my torso out of my hips. An even more important result has been a more relaxed diaphragm. By learning to pull the abdominals in and up, breathing while exercising has become deeper as the diaphragm relaxes. Clearly this yields improved sports performance.

So, let's try it.

Exercise 1 Belly-Breathing

Change into something comfortable, then lie on your back on the floor, or another hard surface, and put your rolled towel or pillow under your knees.

Extend your arms out from your shoulders and relax the backs of your hands on the floor (Illustration 10). Close your eyes and envision your diaphragm and the deep abdominal muscles. Inhale deeply through your nose and pull the air down into your midsection. When you exhale through your nose, feel your midsection pull in (Illustration 8). If your chest is expanding and you're pulling *in* your belly on the inhale, then you are reverse breathing. Keep practicing until you feel

Illustration 8

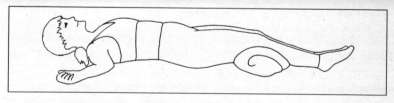

Illustration 9

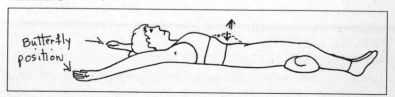

Illustration 10

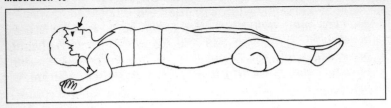

Illustration 11

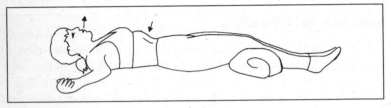

Belly Breathing

the difference. While you are practicing, you will be giving your body a healthy dose of oxygen, so you'll feel more and more relaxed. The more relaxed you become the easier these exercises will be.

Exercise 2 Active Belly Breathing

Lying in the same position, start to lengthen and slow down both your inhalation and your exhalation. Breathe comfortably through your nose and keep your chest and shoulders relaxed. Slowly begin to pull in your abdomen actively as you exhale. *Don't force the length of your breath;* allow your body to establish its own rhythm. As you feel yourself becoming more relaxed and breathing more easily, intensify the pulling in on the exhale. Continue this for a few minutes, *feeling* the elasticity in the muscle fibers and focusing on the active pulling in with each exhale.

Imagine you have a string attached to the inside of your belly button. Pull it all the way back to your spine as you exhale. Completely relax your abdomen on the inhale. Make sure you are breathing through your nose, not your mouth.

Nose breathing has been linked to the parasympathetic nervous system and the relaxation response. Although exhaling slowly through your mouth is a good way to release tension and therefore I use it throughout the stretches, continuous mouth breathing tends to stimulate the fight or flight response. This creates tension in the muscles. When you begin to feel fatigue from the effort, return to nonactive belly breathing and completely relax.

If you have trouble feeling which muscles you're trying to work, get up slowly (you may be a little lightheaded from all the deep breathing) and practice in front of a mirror. Keep your eyes on your midsection, which should fill up like a balloon when you breathe in. (Be careful not to do it more than three or four times in a row—you may hyperventilate.)

IMPORTANT WORD OF WARNING

Each individual's body responds differently to exercise. If during any of the exercises that follow, even the easiest, you feel pain or discomfort of any kind, *immediately release your contraction.* Adjust your position to one that is comfortable. When the discomfort is gone, experiment with a slightly different position. If you felt your back begin to spasm when your legs were extended over the pillow, try the exercise with your knees bent. If your back still does not stay relaxed, try lying on your side. If that still causes your back to tighten up, do only the nonactive Belly Breathing until your muscles become familiar with these targeted movements and get stronger. These exercises are absolutely safe, but they are asking your muscles to contract. The exercises were designed to be modified or adapted to any individual no matter what his or her physical condition. Simply start slowly, with the belly breathing alone if that's all you can do at first. You can learn these techniques!

✤ *Special Tips*

If you are pregnant or elderly or have a condition such as asthma or emphysema, you may want to do this sitting in a chair. Position yourself firmly on your bottom with your feet flat on the floor. Place your hands on your belly and breathe in deeply.

If you have a hard time filling your lungs with air in this position, sit up tall, on your bottom, lift your chest up out of your hips, and do it until you feel your belly moving out as you draw air into your lungs, then in as you exhale. Check your buttocks and shoulders to make sure they stay relaxed.

Exercise 3 Basic Supine In and Up

Lie flat on your back with a pillow or large rolled towel under your knees. Extend your arms out at a diagonal up from the shoulders and relax the backs of your hands on the floor. Your legs are together over the towel roll or pillow, and your buttocks are relaxed. Inhale deeply through your nose, allowing your midsection to expand (Illustration 12). Exhale through your mouth, forcing out most, but not all, of the air, and pull your abdominals *in and up* (Illustration 13). You may feel a slight rotation of your pelvis move your lower back toward the floor. Do not press your back onto the floor. You want to experience only the natural range of motion. Hold that position, with your buttocks relaxed, and go back to breathing easily through your nose. *Do not* allow your midsection to expand when you inhale. Hold your abdominals **in and up** in a tight contraction, feeling your body sink in under your ribs. Count to ten as you continue to breathe, and increase the contraction in your abdominals. Imagine a string attached to the inside of your belly button. Pull that string back toward your backbone and up under your ribs. *Keep breathing.* At the end of your count of ten, relax and return to deep belly breathing.

Repeat 2 or 3 times, then go on to the next exercise.

Illustration 12

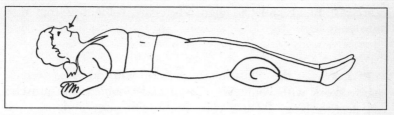

Illustration 13

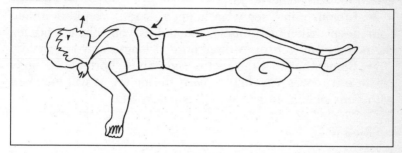

Basic Supine In and Up

✔ Body Check

• *Did you feel your chest drop toward the floor when you relaxed?* You may have been holding a lot of tension in your chest and shoulders. Or were you holding your breath?

If you felt completely out of air after you exhaled, you may have sustained your exhalation too long. Make your exhalation short and fast, pushing the air out of your lungs by blowing out through your mouth as though you were blowing out a candle. (Remember to go back to breathing through your nose.) Don't try to force all the air out of your lungs, just enough to make the pulling in stronger.

• *Did you feel as though your chest pulled down toward your middle when you exhaled?* That's the outer layer of muscle, the rectus abdominis. Focus on the muscles deep inside your body. Your abdomen should *pull in* as you exhale, not flatten.

• *When you relaxed, did you feel your buttocks release?* You may have been doing a pelvic tilt with your buttocks rather than with your abdominals.

These are all natural reactions the first time you do these exercises. Relax and try again. Here are some tips that may help you:

➤ Look at the illustrations before you do the exercise again. Work with your eyes closed and *visualize* the muscles you are working. Picture your body with your abdomen flat and your waist cinched in.

➤ In your mind, see what happens during respiration. See your deep abdominal muscles expand as you inhale, and see them relax and return to their normal length as you exhale.

➤ Remember that the rectus abdominis shortens the body because it moves the chest *toward* the pelvis. It will interfere with your pulling in and up (Illustration 14).

Illustration 14

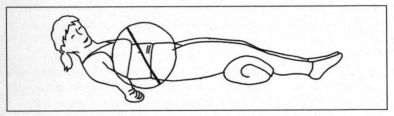

This Move Shortens the Body.

➤ In your mind, *see* and *feel* your body lengthen as you exhale and the muscles pull in and up.

➤ Always return to belly breathing between exercises. This ensures that you are getting a full measure of oxygen and will help you relax so that you don't get too tense during the exercise. The more you practice belly breathing, the more natural it will become. The ability to hold the abdominals in and up and continue to breathe through the nose becomes easier the more relaxed you are during the exercise.

➤ Keep practicing this first exercise until you feel that you are doing it correctly. As long as you belly breathe three or four times between sets, you can't do this exercise too often.

✤ *Special Tips*

If you are pregnant and in your third trimester, you should roll over onto your left side between repetitions. If you can't get down on the floor, you can do this exercise in bed as long as you have a firm mattress. You still need to put a pillow under your knees.

If you have a swaybacked posture (lumbar lordosis), accentuate the rotation of your pelvis by contracting your buttocks; this will assist your lower back to move toward the floor. If you have a normal curve or a flat low back, keep your buttocks relaxed.

Exercise 4 In and Up on Hands and Knees

This is a real strength move. In this position you are working against gravity. All the weight of your organs, body fluids, and tissue in your lower trunk is pressing down against your abdominal wall. When you pull in and up, you are actually lifting the weight of your abdominal contents with those deep abdominal muscles.

Position your body on your hands and knees on the floor (Illustration 15). Find a comfortable neutral position for your back. Is it relaxed? Wiggle your hips (Illustrations 16 and 17). Return to neutral. You want to maintain your own natural curve in the small of your back, so make sure it is not unnaturally flattened.

You should be looking at the floor so that you can keep your head and neck in line with your back. Hold that position. Without allowing the position of your back to change, inhale through your nose into your belly and allow your midsection to expand (Illustration 18). (It feels difficult in this position.) Exhale through your mouth and pull your abdominals **in and up.** Do not allow your back to move (Illustration 19). Now, hold your abdominals in a tight contraction, and breathe in and out through your nose. As you did in the Basic Supine In and Up, you want your breath to be slow and small. At the end of a count of ten, relax and notice whether your back moves.

Sit back on your haunches, relax, and do two or three full

Illustration 15

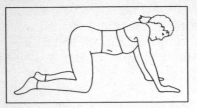

In and Up on Hands and Knees.

Illustration 16

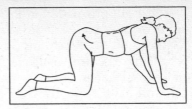

Relax belly.

Illustration 17

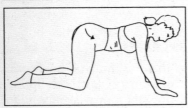

Find neutral with back.

Illustration 18

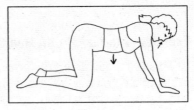

Inhale—expand belly.

Illustration 19

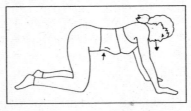

Exhale—lift belly in and up. Hold for count of ten.

belly breaths. Then return to your starting position for the next repetition.

Repeat 2 times, then go on to the next exercise.

✔ *Body Check*

• *Did your back or chest drop when you relaxed?* You may have been tensing up in those areas and rounded your back.

• *Did you have a difficult time breathing in this position?* If so, don't hold the muscles in and up for a full count of ten. Start with a count of three or four. As you get stronger and more accustomed to belly breathing, you will be able to hold the position longer and longer. Go at your own pace.

• *Did you feel a lot of tension (a pulling sensation) just above the small of your back?* This is natural. The transversus abdominis and the obliques are attached to the ribs in the back as well as the front. As you lift and tighten the muscle fibers in your abdomen, you will feel tension in your back as the muscles shorten. The key is to focus on the muscles in the front while holding your back steady.

• *Did you get a crick in your neck?* You may have lifted your head, either to look at yourself in the mirror or just when you were trying to breathe. It is important to keep your head in line with your back while doing the exercise.

Repeat the same visualization techniques you used during the Supine In and Up exercise. Don't repeat this exercise more than two or three times in a row. You may get a little lightheaded. Remember to belly breathe three or four times between sets and to move slowly as you start to return to a standing position.

It's important not to skip steps in any of these exercises. If you do you are likely to compromise your body position. Plus, doing the exercises step by step helps you to remember important points—keeping your head and back in line and breathing.

✤ *Special Tips*

If you can't get down on your hands and knees or have problems with your wrists, use a table or a bench and lean over, resting some of your weight on your forearms. The kitchen counter or sink is a good place (Illustration 20). If you are standing, make sure your knees are softly bent, not locked. If the surface you are leaning over is not low enough for your back to be level, find a comfortable, relaxed position you can hold while you pull your abdominals **in and up.** *Don't allow your back to become round.* Make sure you belly-breathe between sets and move slowly when you stand up straight so you don't get lightheaded.

This next exercise is important because it is applies the in-and-up move to normal standing posture. This is the ultimate goal of these exercises—being able to hold your abdominals

Illustration 20

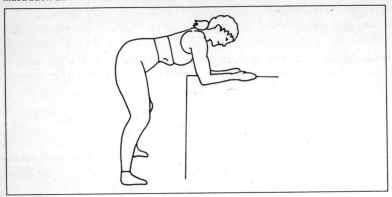

Using Support for Exercise

in and up to keep your body well supported when you're standing and moving normally.

Exercise 5 Standing Forced Expiration of Breath

Stand in front of a mirror in a relaxed position with your feet about 12 to 15 inches apart. Balance your weight evenly. Your knees need to be soft, not locked. Lift your chest up by lengthening the distance between the bottom ribs and your hips (Illustration 21). Your back is lengthened, but relaxed. Make sure you don't tuck your pelvis under. You want to retain the natural curve in the small of your back. Now, keeping your chest raised, relax your shoulders. Inhale deeply through your nose and allow your midsection to expand (Illustration 22). Exhale your breath in a strong, fast expiration through your mouth and pull your abdominals **in and up.** You want the movement to be in your diaphragm and abdominal area, not in your chest and shoulders (Illustration 23). Hold your body stable during expiration, and do not allow your pelvis to jerk under or change position. The move is meant to isolate your abdominals and not involve your buttocks or back. Hold your abdominals in and up and return to

breathing through your nose. Slowly count to ten. Relax and return to the starting position.
Repeat 2 or 3 times, then rest.

Illustration 21   Illustration 22   Illustration 23

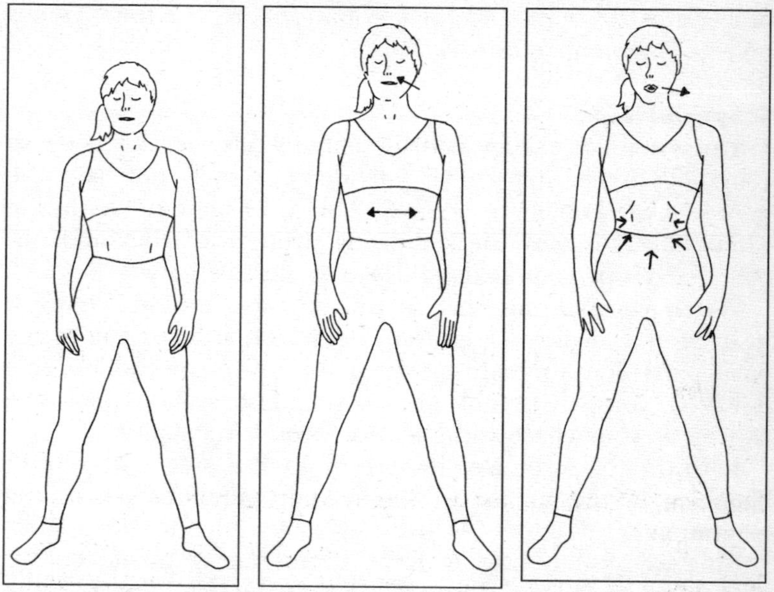

Standing Forced Expiration of Breath

✔ *Body Check*
   • *Did your chest rise up and your belly pull in as you inhaled?* If so, then you were breathing into your chest rather than belly.
   • *Did your body feel as though it shortened rather than lengthened as you exhaled?* If so, you may have involuntarily contracted the rectus abdominis or tucked your pelvis under as you forced the air out.
   • *Did your shoulders feel unnaturally tensed up toward your neck?* After you exhale, do a body check to see where you feel tension. Wherever you find it, let go of it. The only tension you feel should be in your abdominals.
   • *Check your knees right now. Are they locked back, or*

still in a soft bend? This is another place to look when you
do your body check.

• *Did you hold your breath rather than return to slow,
small breathing through the nose?* If you had a difficult time
breathing and holding your abdominals in and up, repeat the
procedure and only hold for a count of three or four (versus
ten) and remember to *breathe!*

✤ Special Tips

The dynamics change considerably in this exercise because
your body is bearing weight (standing). You do not have the
floor as a fixed object to help you hold your body stable during
expiration. It is only the stabilizing strength of your abdominals that keeps your body still as you do this move.

Watch yourself carefully as you do this exercise. Doing it
in front of a mirror is important because that helps you to see
what parts of your body move. If you are comfortable doing
it naked, you will be able to see your entire abdominal area
as well as your chest and back to check for stability.

Perform this exercise, then turn to the side and repeat,
checking in the mirror to see if your pelvis moves during
expiration.

This exercise is also a great stress management tool. It
allows you to "blow off steam" during the day. Try it in the
bathroom while you are brushing your teeth. (Make sure your
mouth is not full of toothpaste when you exhale!)

If a particular condition (pregnancy, advanced age, asthma,
etc.) makes it difficult for you to do this exercise standing,
you may do it sitting down. Find a firm, straight-backed chair
and position yourself firmly on your buttocks with both feet
flat on the floor. Lift your chest up out of your hips, relax
your shoulders and buttocks, and do the exercise. Turn and
sit sideways in the chair and watch for movement in your back
and pelvis in the mirror, just as you would if you were
standing.

These are the basic, most beginning level of the abdominal
exercises. They are effective by themselves or in combination.
To begin the program, do two or three repetitions of each

exercise in the order they appear in this chapter. If three repetitions are too many and you feel lightheaded or short of breath, start with two of each. The easiest combination is the Supine In and Up exercise and the In and Up on Hands and Knees. If you are going to do the first exercise in bed, then get down on the floor for the second exercise. Forced Expiration of Breath can be done anytime throughout the day, but first thing in the morning and last thing at night are convenient times, because if you're like me you're usually in the bedroom or bathroom in front of a mirror. The most important safety tip is to belly-breathe between repetitions, and *go at your own pace.*

Do these twice a day for one week before moving on to the next chapter. By the end of that time you should already start to feel a difference in the way you stand and breathe and in your ability to hold your tummy in.

Don't be in a hurry to move on. If you are having difficulty with the techniques described above, ask a friend to spot check your body position. You are beginning a program of core strength and stability that will stay with you the rest of your life, so take the time to do each move correctly.

My clients range in age from their twenties to their sixties, but they all delight in the simplicity and effectiveness of the program. This letter speaks for itself:

I am twenty-eight years old, and the youngest student in Nancy's class. Yet to my surprise (and everyone else's) my abdominals were the weakest! So weak that I have been unable to do some of the exercises. It's amazing to me that an exercise so simple, easy, and natural really works. I can do this exercise anywhere and at any time of the day.

A registered nurse who has been doing the exercises for several years reports:

I faithfully practice the abdominals every morning before getting out of bed. They have strengthened not only my abdominals, but also my back and improved my posture. I recommend them to patients to do post-op. No more waiting six weeks to get back in shape.

I love the next two letters.

> *On May 14th I had an operation to remove my gallbladder. After the operation, my doctor told me my deep abdominals were more developed than he was used to seeing. I resumed doing the abdominal exercises ten days later. My feeling is that the exercises are the reason for my good condition and my fast recovery from the operation.*

It's not just my clients, but also their doctors who comment on the program's success. One general surgeon wrote me:

> *I recently peformed surgery on a sixty-one-year-old gentleman and noted how firm his abdominal wall appeared. When I asked him about his good condition, he attributed it to your exercise program. His recovery was speedy and he couldn't wait to get back to his exercises!*

Playing Both Ends Against the Middle

Although I have discussed the abdominal cavity—in which the diaphragm forms the roof, and the abdominal muscles the walls—I haven't described the pelvic floor. The term "pelvic floor" is actually a misnomer. It is not an inflexible platform, but rather a very elastic group of muscles that act as a trampoline, expanding and contracting. They support the uterus, the prostate, and the bladder. (I discuss the different types of muscle fibers that comprise the pelvic floor in chapter 5.) Some of those fibers are in a constant state of contraction, lifting and supporting the organs in the abdominal cavity. They play a major role in the release of urine from the bladder. Weakness of these muscles can result in incontinence, reduced sexual function and enjoyment, and prolapse of the organs in that area.

Research has established that specific exercises can restore these muscles to their healthy tone and function. When you are doing the abdominal exercises, concentrate on lifting the pelvic floor **up,** as you do the **in and up** move. Think of a chamber with four walls, a top, and a bottom. Think of pulling the walls in and lifting the bottom up. If you are a woman, imagine you are drawing an object up the vaginal tunnel with suction. Then hold it there. Use your imagination. Don't let a false sense of modesty inhibit you. We are talking about health here. These exercises are important for maintaining circulation and muscle tone in these muscles for both men and women.

And there is more. I teach the abdominal exercises in a series of eight classes, several times a year, under the name "Phenomenal Abdominals." I received this letter from a married couple. The wife had been one of my most enthusiastic students:

> *After fourteen years of marriage, your abdominal and pelvis exercises have certainly brought a new level of excitement into our lives. Long live Phenomenal Abdominals . . . and all their fringe benefits.*

Need I say more?

3

Passive Resistance

You made it! You have completed the first step in the program and done a great job. Let's increase the intensity by adding resistance to the basic Supine In and Up move.

From now on I want you to hold your abdominals **in and up** to the point of fatigue. That means you will hold them in until you can't hold them in any longer. When you have to release the tension in your abdominals, do it slowly, don't just let them go. By working your muscles until they're fatigued you'll increase their strength at an accelerated pace.

To add resistance we're going to start moving body parts. When I was doing the biofeedback testing, the R.N. who was monitoring the equipment asked me, "Why do you need to move anything? It's clear that just the pulling in of the abdominal wall works the muscles effectively." I explained that the reason we add movement is because we move in our normal, everyday activity. The ability to hold the muscles in while we are moving is the *functional application* of these exercises. Providing support for our back during our normal activities is necessary to protect ourselves from injury. Holding the abdominals in while we are moving is the ultimate test of strength for these muscles.

Movement of the arms as you hold in your abdominals adds a lot of resistance, because the muscles that are attached to the rib cage are also attached to the upper arm. (Remember chapter 1?) As your arms move away from the center of your body, there is a pull on the rib cage away from the pelvis. (Put one hand on the bottom of your ribs and move your other arm up over your head and back down. Feel those ribs moving?) If you are lying on your back as you do this, your back will start to arch up off the floor.

Holding your abdominals in and up tightly as you do this stabilizes the rib cage in relation to the pelvis and holds your back down on the floor. This makes your abdominal muscles work harder than before. Let's try it. (Remember, read through each exercise first so you don't skip any steps.)

Exercise 6 Butterfly Arm Move

Lie on your back with a rolled towel or pillow under your knees, and place your arms out in the butterfly stretch (diagonal up from the shoulders). Relax the backs of your hands on the floor, palms up (Illustration 24). Belly-breathe and visualize your abdominal "corset" for a moment. When you are relaxed, **inhale deeply through your nose allowing your midsection to expand. Exhale through your mouth and pull your abdominals in and up.** Go back to breathing easily through your nose. Bend your elbows so that your fingers point toward the top of your head (Illustration 25), and **slowly** begin to *slide* your arms along the floor up over your head, toward each other. Relax the muscles in your shoulder and chest area and keep your arms on the floor for as long as you can (Illustration 26). *Do not allow your back to lift up off the floor.*

Hold your body firmly in place by pulling in and up on

Illustration 24

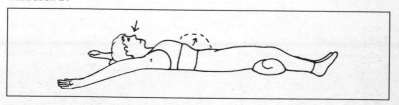

Butterfly Arm Move. Inhale—let belly expand.

Illustration 25

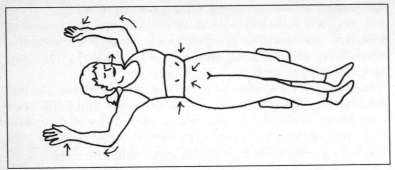

Exhale—pull in and up, bend elbows.

Illustration 26

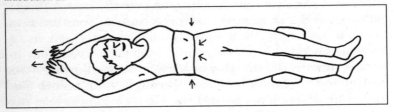

Slide arms upward. Keep back on floor.

your abdominals. When your arms reach their full range of motion, go back and check the rest of your body. Notice where you feel tension and concentrate on relaxing that area. Slow spread your arms open and slide them down into the butterfly position. Release your abdominals slowly and return to belly-breathing.

Repeat 1 time, then go on to the next exercise.

✔ *Body Check*
• *Did you feel a lot of tension in the top of your shoulders and at the base of your neck as you slid your arms over your head?* That's natural. The muscles that elevate the shoulder area are working to move your arms above your head.

When you feel the tension building up, stop your arms

where they are and *consciously* relax that area. As you feel the tension release, continue sliding your arms up.

If you have a history of shoulder injury or have restricted motion in your shoulders, only slide up as far as it feels comfortable. *Do not force the arms to move upward if you feel pain or discomfort.*

• *Did the back of your arms or elbows lift off the floor as you began to move them up?* The muscles that bring the arms down to the body will be in a stretched position as you slide your arms up over your head. Pay close attention to what you feel in your upper body. This exercise is an excellent way to discover areas of muscle tightness and imbalance in your body. The more you do of this program of exercises and moving stretches, the stronger and more flexible your body will become.

If any movement of your arms upward causes you discomfort, skip this exercise and move on to the next one.

❖ *Special Tips*

If the tension in your neck or shoulder areas is too uncomfortable, slide one arm over your head at a time, then slide them back down together. If even this is not possible, slide one arm up and back down and then move the other arm likewise.

Exercise 7 Angels in the Snow

While on your back with your arms in the butterfly stretch, allow your arms to feel very heavy and sink into the floor (Illustration 27). **Inhale deeply and allow your midsection to expand. Exhale, and pull your abdominals in and up. Gently curl your pubic bone up toward your chest, mov-**

Illustration 27

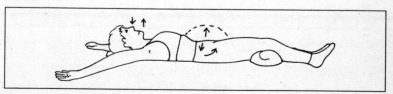

**ing your body into a pelvic tilt. Slowly begin to slide one
arm up by your head as the other arm slides down next
to your hip** (Illustrations 28 and 29). *Keep the arms on the
floor, fully extended with palms up, throughout the movement.*
Do not pause when you reach the end of your range of motion; immediately begin to slide both arms in the opposite
direction. Keep the motion going for ten or twelve slides,
keeping your abdominals in and up and holding your back in
a stable position. Hold your body very still as you move the
arms, and don't allow your back to lift off of the floor. *Remember to keep your arms on the floor.* Allow them to drag as you
slide them up and down, only going as far as it feels comfortable. When you have completed the slides, return to your
butterfly position and rest.

Illustration 28

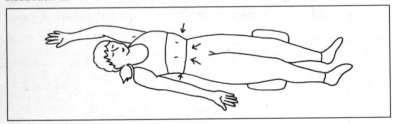

Illustration 29

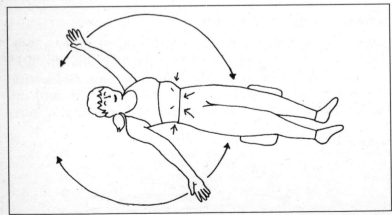

Angels in the Snow

✣ *Special Tips*

The Angels in the Snow exercise and the Alternate Arm Move, which follows, are double duty exercises. They also appear in the next chapter as range of motion exercises. In this chapter, as abdominal exercises, they are still actually working the back. You will feel the muscles between the shoulder blades as they assist and stabilize the arm movement. In the Angels in the Snow, the key is to let the arms drag. Don't use any muscles to *lift*. Only use muscles to *pull*. If you have any restriction in your shoulder area, modify the move to stay within a range that is comfortable and pain free.

The next exercise takes a bit longer than most in the program, but stick with it, you'll be glad you did.

Exercise 8 Alternate Arm Move

After you have completed the previous exercise, do not release your abdominals. Continue to breathe comfortably, holding your abdominals in and up. Feel how your weight is distributed on the back of your ribs. Notice if the small of your back is touching the floor. **Slowly slide your right arm and bring it down until your hand is resting next to the side of your thigh. Turn the palm down. Keep your arm fully extended and close to your body. Then slide your extended left arm until it is next to the side of your head with the palm facing up.** *Do not bend your arm.* **Holding your abdominals in and up in a tight contraction, slowly begin to lift your arms over the top of the body, alternating their positions** (Illustration 30).

Illustration 30

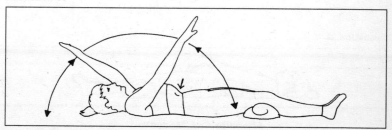

Focus on moving your arms at the same pace. Repeat again in the opposite direction. Keep your arms in motion, not stopping when you reach the end of your range. Immediately begin the move back in the opposite direction. You hold your back and ribs motionless during the arm sweep by pulling **in and up** with your abdominals. Continue to move the arms slowly until you have completed five or six sweeps. Breathe easily through your nose and relax the rest of your body (that's the hard part). At the end of the last sweep, allow both arms to meet over the center of your chest with your fingers pointed toward the ceiling (Illustration 31). Slowly lower them back over your head until your fingers brush the floor (Illustration 32). Lift them back up and move them toward your feet until your fingertips are resting lightly on your thighs (Illustration

Illustration 31

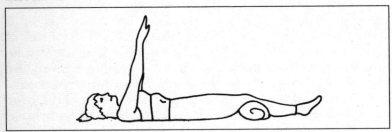

Illustration 32

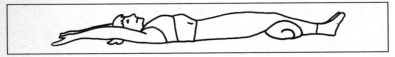

Illustration 33

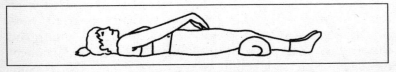

Alternate Arm Movement

33), then lift and return them to the center of your chest. Pulling in tightly on your abdominals, open your arms out and slowly lower into your butterfly position. Keep your abdominals in and up and relax the rest of your body. Breathe easily for a moment, then slowly release and return to belly-breathing.

This exercise takes about 8 minutes. You only need to do 1 repetition.

✤ Special Tips

If getting down on the floor is difficult for you, you can perform the two previous exercises while sitting in a chair. If you are in your third trimester of pregnancy, roll over onto your left side and belly-breathe for a few moments between these three exercises. Then resume your exercise position and proceed.

Exercise 9 Standing Alternate Arm Move

If it's convenient, you should stand in front of a mirror as you do this exercise. If you can't, simply focus on feeling your body position. This is also a long exercise.

Stand with your feet hip width apart and your arms at your side. Relax your shoulders and think about lengthening your spine. Inhale deeply through your nose and allow your midsection to expand. Exhale through your mouth, and pull your abdominals **in and up** (Illustration 34).

Notice your rib cage in the mirror. Your goal is to hold your trunk very still as you move your arms. Holding your abdominals **in and up in** a tight contraction, raise your arms to shoulder height, palms facing forward (Illustration 35). Begin to move your arms as you did in the Angels in the Snow exercise. **Slowly move your left arm up toward your head as you bring your right arm down next to your hip** (Illustration 36). **Keep the motion going, reversing the movement.** Keep your arms moving. (If your shoulder movement is limited, stay within the range of motion that is comfortable.) Focus on moving your arms at the same pace.

Illustration 34

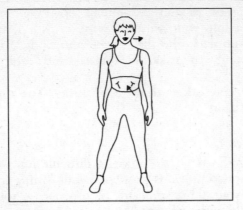

Illustration 35

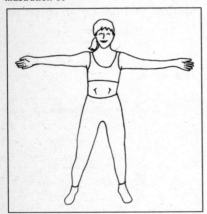

Illustration 36

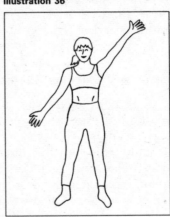

Standing Alternate Arm Movement. Sweep at sides six times.

Repeat the movement 6 times, keeping continuous motion with your arms.

Do not allow the position of your back or rib cage to change. After your sixth move, allow the arms to stay where they are, one up by your head, one down by your hip (Illustration 37). **Begin to sweep your arms, as in the Alternate Arm Move, over the front of your body** (Illustration 38). **Breathing easily through your nose, sweep your arms 6**

Illustration 37

Illustration 38

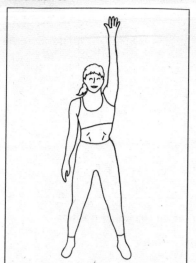
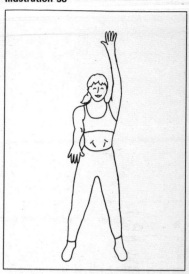

Sweep over front six times.

times and pull in on the strings of your abdominal corset. **At the end of your last sweep, allow both arms to
meet at the center of your chest, then open them out
to chest level** (Illustration 39). **Bring right arm across to
touch the front of your left arm** (Illustration 40). Repeat
with other arm. Slowly lower your arms into a relaxed position.
Now check the rest of your body and relax any tension in
your neck or shoulders. Keep your abdominals **in and up**
to the point of fatigue, then **slowly** release and return to
belly breathing.
   Do only 1.

✤ *Special Tips*

   You'll be working the same muscles whether you sweep your
arms as I've described above, or use some invention of your
own. The point is to move the arms continuously while you
maintain the stability of the middle of your body. Keep the
motion going for as long as you can while keeping the abdomi-

Illustration 39 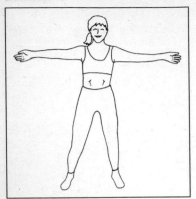 **Illustration 40**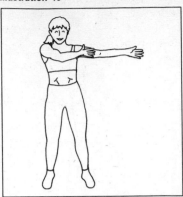

Repeat with other arm and return to resting position.

nals tightly pulled in and up. Be aware of any tension you are holding in your shoulders. That's one of the most common problems I see in my clients. Keep your neck and shoulders as relaxed as you can.

TAKE A BREAK AND REST. YOU DESERVE IT!

The next two exercises are variations of the Active Belly Breathing described in chapter 2. I've included them here because you can easily add an element of resistance to the basic exercise by changing your position, which makes pulling in and up more difficult. When you are lying on your side or facedown, gravity pulls on your abdominal contents. In either position they are out of the pelvic cavity and lying against the abdominal wall, so you are actually lifting weight just as you did with the In and Up on Hands and Knees. These positions are an intense and efficient method of strengthening the abdominal wall. If you have a *firm* mattress these can be done in bed.

Do this combination when you wake up, and you'll send the message to the abdominal muscles that will establish a pattern of muscular function for the entire day. Do it at night when you get into bed. It will fatigue the abdominal muscles and relax you before you fall asleep. The Side-Lying Active In and Up is also important practice for one of the most difficult exercises in the program.

Exercise 10 Side-Lying Active In and Up

Lie on your side with your head supported on your arm or on a pillow, and pull your knees up into a 90-degree bend (Illustration 41). Your head, neck, and spine should be in alignment. Begin to belly-breathe deeply through your nose, focusing on the abdominal wall, moving out as you inhale and moving in as you exhale. Your belly is relaxed. *Feel* the weight of your abdominal contents lying upon the inside of your abdominal wall closest to the floor. **Begin to focus on actively stretching your abdominals as you inhale** (Illustration 42) **and actively pulling in as you exhale** (Illustration 43). Breathe this way for a few minutes, sustaining your exhalation as long as is comfortable and **pulling** deeply into the body.

After each sustained exhale, inhale deeply and allow the belly to stretch (but stay relaxed!). Continue to breathe this way and begin to actively lift the abdominal contents back into the pelvic cavity as you exhale and pull in. *Feel* the muscles working and continue this exercise until your abdominals begin to feel fatigued. After one more deep inhalation, exhale, pull **in and up,** and hold to the point of fatigue. Release the tension in the abdominal wall and return to relaxed belly breathing. **Immediately go on to the next exercise.**

IMPORTANT WORD OF WARNING

If you are in your third trimester of pregnancy, skip the next exercise. Turn to the other side and repeat the Side-Lying In and Up. If you are uncomfortable lying on your right side for even a short time, do this exercise only on your left side.

Illustration 41

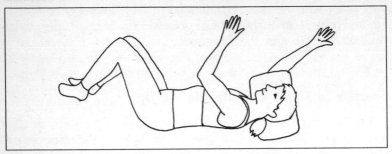

Illustration 42

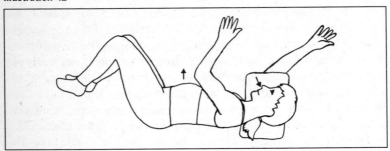

Illustration 43

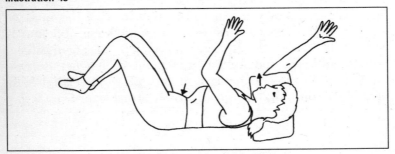

Side-Lying Active In and Up

Exercise 11 Prone Active In and Up

Lie on your stomach with your forehead resting on the back of your hands. Your legs should be about 12 inches apart. Adjust your position so that your pelvic area opens and your lower back is relaxed (Illustration 44). Begin to belly-breathe deeply, focusing on the abdominal wall moving out as you inhale, and *actively* lifting the abdominal contents back into the pelvic cavity as you exhale and pull **in and up** (Illustration 45). After each sustained exhalation, inhale deeply and allow the belly to stretch. Breathe this way several times, then pull your abdominals in and up and hold to the point of fatigue (Illustration 46). Release and return to relaxed belly breathing.

Illustration 44

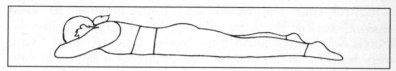

Illustration 45

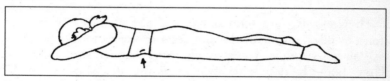

Illustration 46

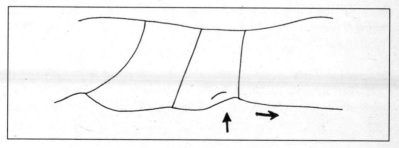

Prone Active In and Up

Now we're going to increase the resistance by adding movement of the legs. Let me tell you a little secret: All those years we were doing leg lifts were a waste of time. The abdominal muscles are not attached to your legs. The muscles in the legs are not attached to your abdomen. So movement of the legs themselves cannot strengthen the abdominals. It's anatomically impossible.

Stabilization of the pelvis while you move the legs is what strengthens the abdominal muscles. Remember, the action of the deep abdominals is to stabilize the pelvis in relation to the rib cage. In other words, they hold the body in correct alignment. Because the muscles in the legs are attached to the pelvis, moving the legs alters the position of the pelvis, and this creates resistance against which to work the abdominals.

When you lie on your back with your knees bent, you have rotated the pelvis and shortened the abdominal area between your belly button and your pubic bone. (Try it and see.) **As you pull your abdominals in, the area shortens even more. Moving the legs away from the body pulls the pelvis downward, causing the abdominal muscles to work very hard to hold the pelvis in its starting position. Stabilization of the pelvis is what strengthens the muscles.**

The following are more advanced abdominals that can be done in place of any of the previous exercises in this chapter. As you get stronger, you may also add them to your program. They should be done only after a few minutes of belly breathing and one Basic Supine In and Up to ensure you are relaxed. Because they are advanced, I advise you not to do them all in one session. Choose one or two and add them to your regular routine.

✤ *Special Tips*
If during any of these exercises you need to rest, release your abdominals between performing the moves on the right and left, then continue.

Exercise 12 Double Heel Slides

Lie on your back, bend your knees, and place your feet on the floor with your arms in the butterfly stretch. The inside of your feet and knees should be close enough to touch for control during this move (Illustration 47). Adjust your body so that your lower back is comfortable. *Feel* how your weight is distributed on the back of your rib cage and your pelvis. **Inhale deeply through your nose, allowing your midsec-**

tion to expand. **Exhale through your mouth and pull your abdominals in and up.** Go back to breathing in and out through your nose and do not allow your midsection to expand. **Creep your toes away from your body (keeping your feet together), extending your legs as far as you can go and still keep your feet flat on the floor** (Illustration 48). *Do not allow the position of your back to lift or change position.* Keep your abdominals in and up. Check the rest of your body. Notice where you feel tension and relax it. **Release the tension in the right calf.** Your toes will lift off the floor but the heel will remain. **Slowly slide your right heel back until your leg is in the bent knee position and your foot is flat on the floor** (Illustration 49). **Repeat with the other leg.** Relax the rest of your body and pull in and up with your abdominals. Hold to the point of fatigue, then slowly release and return to belly breathing.

Do 1 or 2 repetitions.

Illustration 47

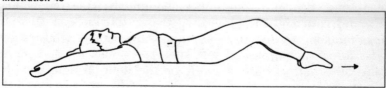

Illustration 48

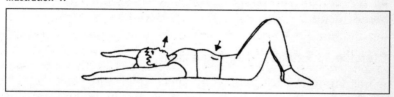

Illustration 49

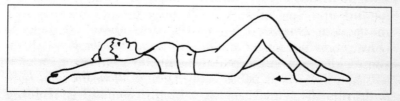

Double Heel Slides

✔ *Body Check*
• *Did you feel wobbly as you were creeping your toes away from your body?* You may not have had your feet and knees together during that part of the move. Keeping contact between your feet and your knees during the move will give you much more control and help you to creep your feet out farther.
• *Did your lower back arch off the floor as your feet were moving out, even though you were holding your abdominals in tightly?* Squeeze your buttocks together and gently rotate your pelvis up while you are doing this exercise. Think about curling your pubic bone up toward your chest. This will help hold your back firmly on the floor. As your abdominals get stronger and you do the moving stretches, it will become easier to keep your body in proper alignment.

❖ *Special Tips*
If you are in your third trimester of pregnancy, do not do the next three exercises. You may substitute Double Heel Slides instead.

Exercise 13 Extended Leg Movement

Lie on your back with your knees bent and your feet flat on the floor. Place your palms on your hip bones, pressing your fingertips into your lower abdominals (Illustration 50). **Extend your right leg level with your left knee.** Feel your legs touching to be sure your thighs are parallel (Illustration 51). Keep your extended left knee soft (relaxed), and make sure both buttocks are squarely on the floor. **Inhale deeply through your nose, and allow your midsection to expand. Exhale through your mouth, and pull your abdominals in and up.** Now breathe easily through your nose. **Slowly move your extended leg to the side about 20 degrees** (Illustration 52). *Keep the other hip firmly on the floor.* When you feel it begin to lift, pull in tightly on your lower abdominals and bring your pelvis level. *Do not allow the bent knee to drop to the side as you move your extended leg.* **Holding your abdominals in a tight contraction, slowly move**

Illustration 50

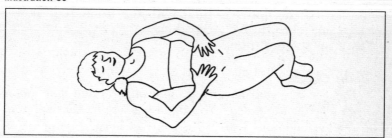

Illustration 51

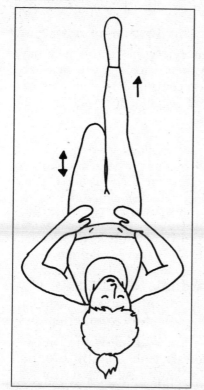

Illustration 52

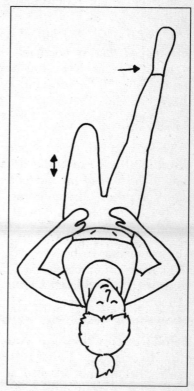

Extended Leg Movement

your left leg back to center, bend the knee, and place your foot on the floor. Repeat with the other leg. Slowly release, and return to belly breathing.

Do 2 or 3 repetitions.

✔ *Body Check*
   • *Did you feel your abdomen bulge slightly and your body shorten when you exhaled?* You don't want to let that happen. The rectus abdominis will try to contract because your leg is lifted and the position of your pelvis is altered. Keep your deep abdominals pulled in and up tightly throughout the move. They will pull the more superficial muscles in with them.
   • *Did you feel the hip of your bent leg lift off the floor as you moved the extended leg out to the side?* You may have gone out too far. Keep the movement small. If you move the leg out only 10 degrees and keep control of your abdominals, that's enough. (Watch your bent leg too, to make sure the knee doesn't lean out to the side.)

These next two exercises are very difficult, so don't attempt them until you can easily do all of the previous ones. *If you have a history of an unstable pelvis or have scoliosis, avoid these exercises.* Straightening out one leg at a time as described below alters the position of the pelvis. This movement could cause you some discomfort. Check with your back health care provider before trying this exercise.

Exercise 14 Single Leg Lower and Lift

Lie on your back with your knees bent and your feet flat on the floor. Your arms start out in the butterfly position. **Inhale deeply through your nose and allow the midsection to expand. Exhale through your mouth and pull your abdominals in and up.** Now breathe easily through your nose. **Extend and lift your right leg up to the level of the left knee** (Illustration 53). Touch the insides of your knees together to make sure they are even and that both hips are firmly on the floor. **Slowly lower your extended leg**

until your heel lightly touches the floor (Illustration 54), but don't let it rest there. Hold your abdominals in and up in a tight contraction and do not allow your back to arch from the floor. **Slowly lift your leg back to the level of the other knee. Bend your knee and place your foot on the floor. Repeat with the left leg.** Slowly release your abdominals and return to belly breathing.

Do 3 or 4 repetitions.

Illustration 53

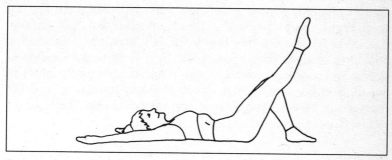

Illustration 54

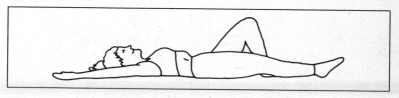

Single Leg Lower and Lift

✔ *Body Check*

• *Did you feel a lot of tension in your upper and midback as you were lowering your leg?* Move your arms to your sides, letting your hands rest on your pelvis as you do the exercise. *Consciously* relax your upper body.

• *Did your back arch off the floor even with your abdominals pulled in as tightly as you could?* You may not be strong enough yet to lower the leg all the way to the floor. Squeeze your buttocks together and rotate your pelvis upward, then only lower your leg halfway before returning it. As your abdominals get stronger you will be able to go all the way down and back up and hold your back stable.

✤ *Special Tips*

If you cannot get down on the floor to do any of the extended leg exercises, try this: Stand next to a countertop or use the back of a chair for support. Standing with your weight evenly balanced on both legs, **inhale deeply through your nose, allowing your midsection to expand. Exhale through your mouth and pull your abdominals in and up tightly. Keeping your left knee soft, lift the right leg up to a right angle from the front of your hip** (Illustration 55). **Slowly extend the leg until it's straight** (Illustration 56). Do not allow your upper body to move down toward your pelvis or your pelvis to tuck under. Hold your abdominals in tightly and keep your back erect. **Bend your knee and return your foot to the floor. Repeat with the other leg.**

Do 3 or 4 repetitions.

Illustration 55

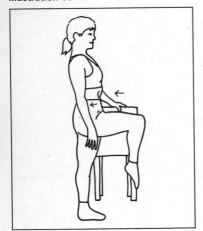

Illustration 56

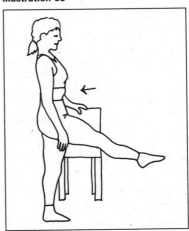

Special Tips for Exercise 14

Exercise 15 Alternate Heel Slides

Lie on your back with your knees bent and feet together. You may place your arms in the butterfly stretch or let your hands rest lightly on your abdomen (Illustration 57). **Inhale deeply, allowing the abdomen to expand, then exhale through your mouth and pull your abdominals in and up.** Focus on pulling in the lower abdominals and gently curl your pubic bone up toward your chest. Feel your lower back move toward the floor and maintain that position throughout the exercise. **Keeping your abdominals in and up, slowly slide your right foot out until your leg is fully extended onto the floor** (Illustration 58). **Maintaining this position, slowly slide your left leg out** (Illustration 59). **When both legs are fully extended, begin to slide your right leg back into the bent-knee position. Keeping your abdominals in and up and your back stable, slide your left leg back to starting position.**

Repeat 4 to 6 times.

Illustration 57

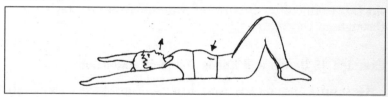

Illustration 58

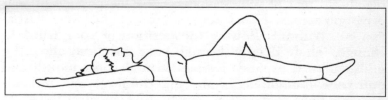

Illustration 59

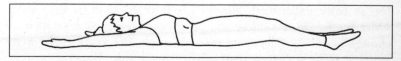

Alternate Heel Slides

✤ *Special Tips*

Even if you have significantly strengthened your abdominals with the previous exercises, you may have a hard time holding your body stable in this one, particularly if you have a strong curve in your lumbar area. Try contracting your buttocks and increasing your pelvic tilt. If you feel your back lifting off the floor, don't attempt to slide your legs all the way out. Just move them as far as you can until you gain the strength to hold your back firmly against the floor.

This next exercise sounds difficult because there is so much to concentrate on. It's been a standard rehabilitative exercise prescribed by physical therapists for stretching and strengthening the back. It has not been traditionally grouped with abdominal exercises despite its clear benefits. This a great abdominal strengthener because you're working against gravity, and if performed regularly, it will improve your balance immensely.

Having a friend check your body alignment is very helpful, since it's difficult at first to tell whether you are staying level throughout the move.

Exercise 16 Hands and Knees Diagonal Extension

Get on your hands and knees. Your knees should be directly under your hips and your hands on the floor just slightly in front of your shoulders. *Feel* the position of your pelvis, rib cage, and head. You want them to be level (Illustration 60). **Without allowing the position of your trunk to change, inhale deeply through your nose and allow the midsection to expand. Exhale through your mouth and pull your abdominals in and up. Holding your abdominals in a tight contraction, slowly slide your left leg back, keeping your toes on the floor** (Illustration 61). **When your leg is fully extended, slowly lift it until it is in line with your back.** *Do not allow the position of your back or hips to change or rotate* (Illustration 62). **Slowly lift your right arm until it is in a direct line with your back** (Illustration 63). *Do not lift your head.* Keep your abdominals in and up and

Illustration 60

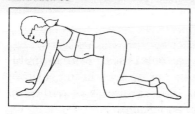

Illustration 61

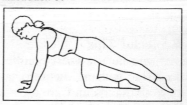

Illustration 62

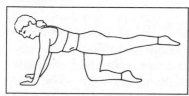

Illustration 63

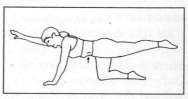

Hands and Knees Diagnoal Extension

breathe through your nose. **Slowly lower your arm and return your hand to the floor. Slowly lower your leg until your toe touches the floor and return it to its starting position.** Hold your back and pelvis level, and *keep your abdominals in and up.* **Repeat with your left arm and right leg.** After completing both sides, release your abdominals, sit back, and relax.

Do 1 repetition only.

✔ *Body Check*

• *Did you feel wobbly as soon as you lifted your extended leg?* You may have had your legs closer together than your arms when you began. The arms and legs need to be the same width apart to provide support for the body as you lift your leg.

• *Did you feel a crick in your neck as you extended either leg or your arm?* You may have been holding your neck in extension (chin lifted) rather than allowing the head to stay in line with the back throughout the exercise. If you can, do this in front of a floor-length mirror. Position your body parallel to the mirror, keep the head in line with the back, and look over your shoulder so that you can observe yourself without straining your neck.

✤ Special Tips

If you have a wrist condition, or any other physical limitations that make it uncomfortable or unsafe for you to get down on your hands and knees, adapt the exercise as described in Exercise 4, In and Up on hands and Knees.

You have just completed a series of unique abdominal exercises (not a crunch in the bunch!). You have been introduced to muscles you may not have known you had. You have learned that slower, smaller, and more controlled is a safer and more effective way to strengthen the body. You have learned the process of isolation, both in contraction of specific muscles and in relaxation. By this time you should have discovered that you can feel relaxed and refreshed after doing your abdominal exercises, rather than fatigued and sweaty, with an aching lower back or neck.

So if you are still doing any form of sit-up, curl-up, crunch, or leg lift, I urge you to "go with haste" to the next chapter and change your workout.

4

Crunching the Numbers

It's 7:00 A.M. You've just awakened, gone into the bathroom, and you see yourself in the mirror. The image you see has a protruding abdomen and slumped shoulders. You already look tired, even though you've just gotten out of bed.

You say to yourself (maybe even out loud), "I've *got* to do something about this belly. I *hate* it." You try to stand up straight and hold your tummy in, but the effort exhausts you. So you go back in the bedroom, get down on the floor, and start to do crunches. The minute you start you can feel the strain on your lower back. After ten you've broken into a sweat and your neck is killing you.

You stop and get up off the floor, thinking, *I can't do this now, I'll be late for work. I'll do them when I get home.* Now you're more exhausted than you were before, and you feel irritated and slightly depressed. Sound familiar?

Let's try another scenario.

It's 7:00 A.M. You wake up and stretch, rolling over onto your back. You reach up, pull your pillow down, and put it under your knees. You're rested and relaxed after your night's sleep, but you take a moment and breathe fully and deeply. You do a strong exhale, pull your abdominals in, and hold them in firmly while you allow the rest of your body to stay relaxed. You concentrate on feeling your body and the new strength in your abdomen. You use your hand to feel your belly and it's pulled in and firm. You hold until you feel fatigue in your abdominal muscles, then you slowly release and stretch again. You get out of bed and get down on the floor on your hands and knees, do three repetitions of In and Up on Hands and Knees, and then stand up, feeling energized and good about yourself.

You go into the bathroom and look in the mirror. The image you see is lengthened, relaxed, and well supported. You notice you're standing taller than you used to and even if you have some extra fat on your belly, it looks firm and pulled in. You do a Standing Forced Expiration of Breath and see the muscles pull in even more, You like what you see, so you smile at yourself as you pick up your toothbrush. It's now 7:15.

Sound appealing? This *can* be the beginning of your day, every day.

Below the Belt

The days of doing three or four sets of twenty-five crunches are over. The days of strengthening your abdominals all through the day are here. It's natural, it's functional, and it's possible.

Let's face it. None of us have ever looked forward to doing our crunches, but we did them anyway because we were told they would give us the "rippling abs" and lean look that put the guys and gals on the covers of magazines.

None of us consider that the models have very little body fat. Of course the ripples in their abdomens show. The rectus abdominis is a superficial muscle, and those ripples are intersections where tendons attach the muscle to the layer of fascia underneath. The truth is, those ripples don't do a thing for pulling the belly in *or* providing support for the back.

Unfortunately, advertisers insist on presenting us with role models that bear very little resemblance to the average person. So we have been doing exercises that don't provide us with what we want or need: to look and feel better about our own bodies.

In September 1991 the *Journal of Human Muscle Performance* reported the results of a study completed at the Physical Therapy Department of California State University in Long Beach. The purpose of the study was to determine whether curl-up exercises increased abdominal strength. The test was completed on a group of randomly chosen subjects who went through an abdominal regime of curl-ups, against a control group of people who did not participate in the training. The exercise group was divided into two smaller groups: one performed the exercises with added weight for resistance, the other without. The results were measured by a Kin Com isokinetic dynamometer, which registers muscle force when muscles are moved at a constant speed.

According to the measurements recorded on the Kin Com, neither one of the exercise programs increased the strength of the abdominal muscles significantly. The conclusion of the study was that even though curl-up exercises involve a high level of muscle activity, they do not tax the abdominal muscles enough to result in a measurable increase in strength.

The rectus abdominis and the external obliques are the more superficial layers of abdominal musculature and are the primary muscles we use when doing traditional abdominal exercises. (Traditional abdominal exercises include curl-ups, crunches, leg lifts, knee pull-ups, etc.). These two muscles are used functionally whenever you bend or rotate the body off of its center of gravity. In other words, you use these muscles every day. If you can bend over to pick something up, get up out of bed, or turn your upper body and look over your shoulder, these muscles are functionally strong.

If, when you are standing, your chest is dropped and your abdomen is hanging out, you're actually allowing your abdominal wall to bulge. If your pelvis is rotated so that you are sway-backed, or your pelvis is thrust forward into a flat-back posture, then your deeper layers of abdominal muscles are not functionally strong. In other words, these muscles are not doing what they were designed to do.

The rectus abdominis actually shortens the body when it contracts, because its primary function is to move the upper body toward the pelvis or the pelvis up toward the rib cage. It compresses the space between the bottom ribs and the top of the hips. When in contraction, this muscle creates a taut, slightly protruded outer abdominal wall, the *opposite* of being pulled in. Remember, the ratio of extensors to flexors needs to be one to one-half times. That means the muscles that hold you erect need to be stronger than the muscles that pull you forward. Overstrengthening the rectus abdominis changes that ratio and holds the body in a slightly flexed position all the time.

The Straight and Narrow

Think about this: The average person with poor posture (and that *is* the average person) has shoulders that roll forward and a dropped chest. A good many people want to strengthen their abdominals because when they look in the mirror, they see a protruding abdominal wall. So what do they do? They do traditional abdominal exercises to pull in their abdomen. Here's the bad news: They don't help!

The deeper layers of muscle, the transversus abdominis and the internal obliques, create a firm, *pulled-in* appearance when contracting. They actually *lengthen* the body by increasing the space between the bottom ribs and the top of the hips as they pull inward, lifting and supporting the rib cage. The result is a leaner and more symmetrical look.

When you are standing without muscle support, gravity pulls down and slightly forward on your abdominal contents: They will protrude out of the pelvic bowl. This causes increased strain on the lumbar spine as well as compression on the pelvic floor and the organs in the urogenital system: the kidneys, bladder, testes, prostate, uterus, and ovaries.

The transversus abdominis and the internal obliques compress the abdomen, with all its contents, and line up the rib cage and the pelvis. That is their primary function. This intra-abdominal pressure literally holds the guts in the body and lifts and supports the rib cage on the pelvis, thereby reducing the strain and compression on the spine and internal organs by as much as 50 percent.

You strengthen all of the muscles in the abdominal group when you do the Basic In and Up move or any of the other exercises. The exercises in this chapter all involve more participation by the two superficial layers of muscle, the rectus abdominis and the external obliques, because they involve movement in the pelvis to create resistance. The slight flexion movements are performed with the deeper muscles pulled in tightly throughout the exercises. Because pulling in and up with the internal obliques rotates and fixes the pelvis in place, moving the pelvis causes a lengthening contraction. As discussed in chapter 1, this is the type of contraction that strengthens muscle tissue the most.

When the abdominal wall is pulled inward, the rectus abdominis is actually lengthened; therefore movement of the trunk, which normally involves shortening of this muscle, creates increased resistance. This serves to strengthen the rectus abdominis more than you could with a normal shortening contraction like a crunch or curl-up. Holding the transversus abdominis and the internal obliques in against the pull of the rectus abdominis trying to shorten and push the abdominal wall out is also intense resistance for these deeper muscles.

The stronger you get, the more you will find yourself including the basic moves throughout the day. You will discover you are automatically pulling in every time you pick up a bag of groceries, push the lawn mower, sweep or rake the leaves, or shovel snow. They'll become a part of your life.

Moreover, the EMG testing that I conducted showed that the standing exercises produced an even greater response in the muscles than the ones done lying on the floor. That means that as you begin to integrate these moves into your normal, daily function, you will be actively strengthening your abdominal muscles as you are doing other things, even other exercise.

Imagine being able to go for a power walk, work out on the stair climber, cross country ski, or do other aerobic exercise and know that you have already completed your abdominal workout. No more getting down on the floor when you're already fatigued to pump out those terrible, uncomfortable crunches. If you wish, you *can* get down on the floor, stretch, and finish up with the Basic Supine In and Up, and feel relaxed and refreshed. But if you don't have time, you don't have to. You have already done it!

And best of all, this is a program for everyone, as the following letter shows:

I had been working as a professional ski patrolman for eleven years, an occupation that I loved. Following an injury from a fall, an MRI revealed I had two herniated discs. Anything to do with flexion, sitting in a chair, shoveling snow, putting on ski boots, etc., would bring my back into severe spasms. The daily pain was so bad I considered retiring from the thing I loved most. The conventional abdominal exercises I had been told to do were making me worse. I started Nancy's exercises and started to feel a difference after two weeks. The technique of strengthening the back through the stomach seemed so simple that I was quite skeptical. Now I not only know how to strengthen my abdominals and back, but how to tune in to my body and take measures to maintain my health. I'm thirty-seven years old and still working as a ski patrolman. The daily back pain is gone and I will continue this program forever.

Another client with a back injury rejoiced in a similar recovery:

Five years ago a herniated disc put a severe crimp in my active lifestyle of hiking, biking, golfing, and skiing. I began doing the abdominals and back strengthening exercises and what a difference it has made in my life! I am back doing all the outdoor sports I love and really feel good and more toned then ever before. Even when I am traveling I find myself unconsciously pulling in my abdominal muscles. It has become a way of life. Thankfully from a sixty-three-year-old mountain girl."

Now I know that there will still be a few of you hardcore believers in the "harder is better" or "no pain, no gain" philosophy that still pervades a lot of exercises classes. So, these next exercises should satisfy those of you who still feel you just can't live without crunches. These moves are the *safe* way to perform front trunk flexion: with the deep abdominal wall pulled in.

❖ *Special Tips*

If you are in your third trimester of pregnancy, do not do the exercises in this chapter because of the involvement of the rectus abdominis. Continue to practice the exercises in chapters 2 and 3.

Exercise 17 Hands and Knees with Pelvic Rotation

Get on your hands and knees on the floor. Find a neutral position with your back, and keep your head and neck in line with your spine. **Inhale deeply through your nose and allow your midsection to expand. Exhale through your mouth and pull your abdominals in and up in a tight contraction. Gently rotate your pelvis up toward your chest, allowing the lower back to slightly round** (Illustration 64). Continuing to hold your abdominals in and up, **slowly rotate your pelvis backward and extend the buttocks out and up** (Illustration 65). *Do not arch your back.*

Illustration 64

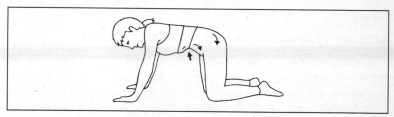

Illustration 65

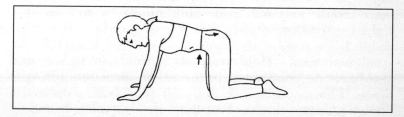

Hands and Knees with Pelvic Rotation

Repeat this pumping motion three or four times slowly, pulling up tightly with your abdominals. Return to your starting position and slowly release your abdominals. Sit back and rest. **Repeat 2 or 3 times.**

✔ *Body Check*
   • *Did you feel strain in your lower back during any part of the exercise?* You may have made the pumping motion too exaggerated and overstretched or overshortened the muscles in the lumbar spine. Keep the move small and controlled. The purpose is not to do full flexion, but to add resistance to the deeper muscles by moving the pelvis toward and away from the rib cage. You want to isolate the movement between your belly button and your pubic bone. If rounding of the back is comfortable but the extension of the hips is not, do only half of the move and come back to neutral with each rotation.

❖ *Special Tips*
   If you are unable to get down on the floor, adapt this exercise by leaning over a table or other surface. Keep your back flat and your knees soft as you pull your abdominals in and up, and proceed with the exercise.

Exercise 18 Supine In and Up with Pelvic Rotation

Lie on your back, bend your knees, and place your feet flat on the floor about 12 inches apart. Your arms are in the butterfly stretch or with your palms resting on your hip bones (Illustration 66). **Inhale deeply through your nose and allow your midsection to fully expand. Exhale through your mouth and pull your abdominals in and up in a tight contraction. Slowly rotate your pelvis, tilting your pubic bone toward the ceiling** (Illustration 67). (This is a *small* movement.) **Hold your abdominals in tightly and slowly rotate your pelvis in the other direction, tilting it down** (Illustration 68). *Do not arch your back.* Repeat this pumping motion three or four times slowly, pulling in and up tightly with your abdominals. Return to your neutral starting

position and hold your abdominals in to the point of fatigue. Slowly release and return to belly breathing.
Repeat 2 or 3 times.

Illustration 66

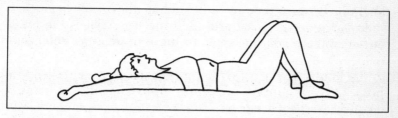

Illustration 67

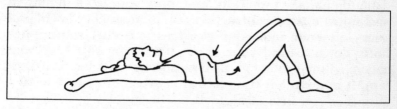

Illustration 68

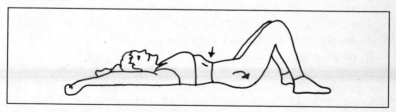

Supine In and Up with Pelvic Rotation

✔ *Body Check*

As in the previous exercise, keeping the movements small and isolated is the key. If you have a tendency toward tight lower back muscles, this exercise may cause you some discomfort. You can modify the exercise by performing the curl-up, then returning your hips to neutral, rather than curling in the opposite direction. If this still bothers your lower back, do not do this exercise.

✤ *Special Tips*
If you are unable to get down on the floor, you may do this exercise sitting in a chair.

Exercises 19 and 20 are the most difficult in the entire program, because they involve holding the trunk motionless while you move both the arms and the legs. This is the maximum resistance you can apply to these muscles as stabilizers.

Exercise 19 Side-Lying In and Up with Curl and Extension

Lie on your right side and support your head on your arm or on a pillow. **Inhale deeply and allow the belly to fully expand. Exhale forcefully and pull your abdominals in and up in a tight contraction** (Illustration 69). **Slowly pull your left knee into your chest as you curl your upper body down toward your knee** (Illustration 70). Keep your abdominals pulled in tightly. **Extend your left leg to its full length and stretch your left arm over your head so that your body is in a straight line** (Illustration 71). *Keep the right knee bent.* Repeat the body curl and extension three or four times, keeping your abdominals pulled in and up. Return to your starting position and slowly release your abdominals. Turn to the other side and repeat.
   Repeat 1 or 2 times.
   If you begin this exercise by practicing your Side-Lying Active In and Up, it will take you several minutes. Then you only need to do 1 repetition on each side.

✔ *Body Check*
   • *Did you feel your belly bulge out as you brought your knee up to your chest?* If so, then your rectus abdominis dominated the move because it is a trunk flexor. It takes enormous control to keep the abdominal wall pulled in during the curl portion of the exercise. Try it again and use your breath as a tool to help hold the deep abdominal muscles in. Breathe in deeply, keeping your abdominals pulled in, *before* you start your curl, and then exhale strongly and pull in even tighter as you draw your knee up. Repeat this breathing process be-

Illustration 69

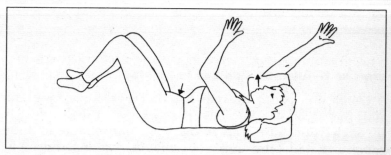

Illustration 70

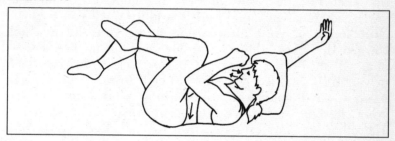

Illustration 71

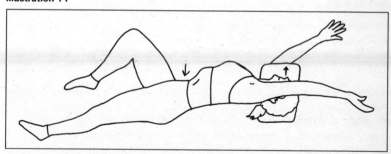

Side-Lying In and Up with Curl and Extension

fore you start the extension. This reinforces the function of the transversus abdominis and the internal obliques and will allow them to pull the rectus abdominis inward along with them.

• *Did you feel some strain in your lower back as you extended your leg?* Then you may have extended your leg too far and arched your back. Be sure you extend the leg only as far as is comfortable as you keep your abdominals pulled in and up.

Exercise 20 Alternate Arm and Leg Move

Lie on your back with your legs over a pillow or towel roll and your arms in the butterfly position. **Inhale deeply through your nose and allow your midsection to fully expand. Exhale through your mouth, forcing most but not all of the air out, and pull your abdominals in and up.** Then breathe easily through your nose. Focus on your lower abdominal area, and **pull in and up until you feel the contraction of your abdominals move your lower back toward the floor** (think of curling your tail up like a scorpion). If you need to, contract your buttocks to increase your pelvic tilt (Illustration 72). **Slowly begin to move your right hand toward your left knee, lifting your knee toward your chest as you move your arm down** (Illustration 73). The other leg stays extended over the roll. Keep your lower

Illustration 72

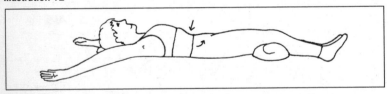

Illustration 73

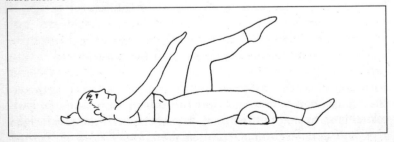

Alternate Arm and Leg Move

back firmly on the floor by increasing the contraction in your abdominals. **Now switch to bring left hand and knee together.** *Continue alternating sides* for eight to ten sweeps, then extend your legs full length over the roll and place your arms in the butterfly stretch. Slowly release your abdominals and return to belly breathing.

Repeat 2 or 3 times or do 1 repetition to fatigue.

✔ *Body Check*
• *Did your belly tighten and bulge out as you brought your knee up to meet your hand?* Use your breath, as you did in the previous exercise, to get the deep abdominal wall pulled in firmly. Move **slowly** but rhythmically as you do this exercise. You will have much better control of your muscles. If you feel any strain in your lower back as you extend either leg back over the roll, you may be allowing your back to arch up off the floor. If you are not able to keep your back firmly against the floor, you may not be ready for this exercise. Go back to whichever leg exercise you do the best and practice! You will get stronger and eventually be able to tackle this one.

The next exercise is just like doing a curl-up or a crunch, but it lets you stand up. It creates no stress or strain on the back or neck, and actually strengthens the bicep (muscle in the upper arm) of the arm you are moving.

Exercise 21 Standing Oblique Crunch

Stand with your feet about hip width apart, keeping your knees soft; do not lock them. With the fingers of your left hand, find your right front hip bone. Now, let that arm just relax by your left side. **Lift your right arm at a 45-degree angle from your body, with the palm of your hand facing you. Make a loose fist** (Illustration 74). **Inhale deeply and allow your abdomen to expand. As you exhale through your mouth and pull your abdominals in and up, pull your right arm down until your elbow touches your right hip bone** (Illustration 75). **Allow your body to curl toward your hip** (Illustration 76). You should feel all the muscles on the right side of your body contracting. **Slowly** stretch back up to your starting position as you inhale. Keep your abdominals in and up throughout the exercise, but each time you crunch down exhale and pull in a little deeper.

Do 8 repetitions, then repeat on the other side. Do 3 sets.

Illustration 74   Illustration 75   Illustration 76

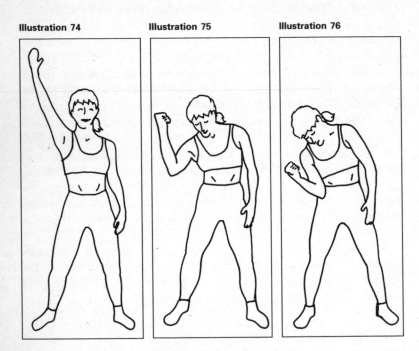

Standing Oblique Crunch

❖ *Special Tips*
If you do this exercise in front of a mirror, you will be able to see the abdominal muscles working. This is a very effective exercise and may be intensified by holding a small hand weight in the extended arm. Some of you may not have a mirror you can work in front of. Although you want to check to see that your palm is facing you, keep your head facing forward as you do the exercise. If you keep your head turned toward your arm, you will overwork a muscle in the neck that rotates your

head to the side. Slowly straighten your arm as you back up. Resist as though you were holding on to something that was pulling you.

So there you have it. A complete abdominal strengthening program that does not include a single sit-up, crunch, leg lift, or any other traditional abdominal exercise. You can strengthen your body *functionally* without stressing or compromising your back or your neck. You're strengthening by *feeling* and *responding* to the messages your body sends you as you exercise. These exercises feel good and help you feel good about yourself, as you take the time to relax and quiet your mind while you work your body.

PART II

Range of Motion Exercises

5

Within Range

How many times did your parents or a teacher tell you to "stand up straight" or "sit up straight"? If your childhood was anything like mine, you heard these messages often. Guess what? Whether your parents knew it or not, they were promoting good health.

In fact, good posture is now considered one of the fundamental signs of being physically fit. Part of the mind-body perspective now accepted by many health care professionals is an understanding of the interconnectedness of all of our physical and psychological parts. This includes the recognition that poor posture has a negative impact on the other systems of the body. I'll explain further later in this chapter.

But what is posture? Kendal and McCreary in *Muscles: Testing and Function* (Williams & Wilkins, 1993) say, "Posture is a composite of the positions of all the joints of the body at any given moment." When someone has poor posture, muscles that are overly shortened hold the body in a position that resists the pull of the muscles that work in opposition to them. This prevents the body from returning to a position of "neutral," or a place of physiological rest. In other words, imbalance in the tension of opposing muscles prevents the body from maintaining a position of good alignment. Poor posture affects all movement, as well as limiting functional flexibility. Good or desirable posture is achieved when the body is in neutral—muscles that work in opposition to one another maintain balance. Equal amounts of tension in opposing muscles allow the body to remain relaxed yet supported.

Pulling Together as a Team

There are about twenty-five or so different muscles that make up what we commonly refer to as back muscles. The back muscles come in three sizes: long, intermediate, and short. The longer muscles are the most superficial or closest to the skin, the intermediate muscles are deeper, and the shortest muscles are right up against the vertebrae.

All of these muscles are actually numerous bundles of muscle fibers that are grouped together and attach to the vertebrae in segments. The longer muscles attach several vertebrae together; the deepest, shortest muscles attach one vertebra to another. This individual attachment allows segmental movement, i.e., flexing or extending only part of the spine at a time. Although when we talk about these muscle fibers we classify them into different groups, in normal movement the muscles work together synergistically.

There are two basic *types* of muscles in the body. These are referred to as postural (tonic) muscles and action (phasic) muscles. The difference between them has to do with the type of fibers they're made of, which are commonly called *slow twitch* and *fast twitch* fibers. The slow twitch fibers have the ability to generate small amounts of force for extended periods because of their ability to draw oxygen from the bloodstream—and oxygen is necessary when doing an activity that requires the muscles to work continuously longer than three or four minutes.

Although we all have some of each type, repetitive activity as well as genetics play a large role in determining what kind of muscles we have. For instance, marathon runners and swimmers usually have a predominance of slow twitch fiber muscles, and their muscles look longer and less bulky, whereas sprinters and weightlifters will have larger, shorter muscles with more fast twitch fibers.

Tonic muscles are made up of slow twitch fibers and are

predominantly the muscles of posture. They basically have *tone*, or some degree of tension in them, whenever you are bearing weight—i.e., when you're sitting or standing. All the deep and intermediate back and neck muscles are examples of tonic muscles. They function continuously and without conscious thought to maintain correct position of the head and spine. Different individual muscles take turns contracting, working in relays. This physiological adaptation keeps them from getting fatigued under normal conditions.

Tonic muscles maintain your body in proper alignment by acting in opposition to one another. For instance, a muscle in the back of the lower leg (the soleus) keeps tension between the heel bone (the calcaneus) and the top of the two bones in the lower leg, the tibia and the fibula. The tension would pull the heel up toward the back of the knee, but is counterbalanced by an opposing pull of the muscles in the front of the leg, the dorsiflexors. These muscles pull the top of the foot up toward the knee. The opposing force between all these muscles holds the leg in proper alignment with the foot.

Phasic muscles, on the other hand, generate large amounts of force for shorter periods of time. Take for example the quadriceps, or muscles in the front of the thigh. These muscles were designed for movement. Their primary action is extension of the knee and flexion of the hip, movements essential to walking or running. Another example of an action muscle is the gluteus maximus. It is the largest muscle in the body and covers the surface of the buttocks. It is the prime mover during any action that involves hip extension, such as walking, skating, or cross-country skiing.

One of the biggest differences between these action and postural muscles is the way they respond to dysfunction or less than normal function. A renowned neurobiologist named Vladamir Janda did research that showed that postural muscles tend to tighten in response to dysfunction or abnormal stress, and action muscles respond by weakening. We can define dysfunction as either lack of use, misuse, or overuse.

Although the action of our muscles is to pull our bones closer together, the body is very efficient at adapting to change or stress; so when a muscle becomes overly tight, the antago-

nist muscle, or muscle that opposes this movement, responds
by weakening and becoming overstretched. This weakening
response is a protection. It prevents our muscles from pulling
the body apart as they compete for domination.

There is a definite correlation between repetitive activity,
functional body strength, and poor or faulty posture. Weakness
from lack of use or tightness of muscles from overuse can
cause poor alignment or posture; just as faulty posture or
alignment can result in stretch weakness and adaptive tightness of specific muscles. Stretch weakness is related to the
amount of time a particular body position allows the muscles
to remain in an elongated position.

To understand how stretch weakness occurs, it helps if you
have a basic understanding of what happens during movement. After a muscle contracts or shortens, it does not sponta-
neously lengthen when you relax. It may release its tension,
but muscular relaxation is passive. It is simply the cessation
of muscle tension, allowing the fibers to return to a neutral
state. The muscle fibers are actually incapable of lengthening
or stretching on their own. The muscles that oppose it (the
antagonist muscles) need to contract or shorten and actually
pull the body back to its original position.

For instance, when the muscles in the chest and front of
the shoulders are continuously held in a shortened position
(in a repetitive activity such as sitting at a computer or driving), there needs to be an equal amount of action by the
opposing muscles to pull the body back into a position of
neutral. Otherwise as the chest muscles become adaptively
shortened, stretch weakness occurs in the muscles in the
upper and midback.

Sticking Your Neck Out

During the evolutionary process, before humans were permanently bipedal and stood erect, the cervical spine was pro-
tected by shoulders that hunched forward and enormously
strong posterior neck muscles. These held the head up against
the pull of gravity, as we walked in a semierect posture like
a gorilla. As we developed fully erect posture, relying less and

less on our arms for support, the huge neck muscles disappeared, atrophying as their function changed. Their job was now to balance the head on top of the spine.

Poor posture affects not only the neck and back, but, as you will learn a little later in the chapter, the shoulders. For example, in the classic faulty posture position known as the forward head, the vertebrae in the middle and lower part of the neck are bent slightly forward, which results in a loss of the normal cervical curve. This creates instability, and puts increased pressure on the cervical discs as the vertebrae are pulled on by the ligaments that hold them together. Eventually significant disc degeneration and arthritis may occur in the neck. Both may be a source of pain and restricted movement.

Because the body requires that the eyes be in the horizontal position in order to maintain equilibrium, the upper part of the neck and head rotate back to accommodate the forward position of the head, creating a kind of "turtle neck" effect. In this position the jaw moves slightly open, changing the bite of the teeth. People with this type of posture usually have rounded shoulders and a depressed chest. When this happens the carotid and vertebral arteries, the spinal cord, and the spinal nerves, all requiring the greatest protection, are potentially compromised.

Although there are different schools of thought about what happens first—head forward or rounded shoulders—I believe that the initial problem is the rounded shoulders. Most of our functional movement (in today's environment) is repetitive and forward oriented. Most of us spend a significant part of the day driving a car, sitting at a desk, and/or working on a computer. As mentioned earlier, in this position, the pectorals, which are the muscles in the chest, as well as the upper trapezius and levator scapula (muscles at the top of the shoulder), become overly shortened and pull the scapula upward and forward. This dramatically changes the biomechanics of the entire shoulder girdle as well as of the neck and cervical spine. The clavicle or collarbone moves forward and down, changing the position of muscles all converging in the shoulder area. It is not uncommon for someone with a forward head and rounded shoulders to have shoulder problems—such as bursi-

tis, or tendonitis. As movement is limited, protecting the in-
flamed area, muscles begin to weaken and rotator cuff
problems may develop.

When the shoulders roll in, and the neck and head pull
forward, the muscles in the middle of the back weaken and
stretch, allowing the shoulder blades to move apart. This results in a rounded upper and middle back. Often the scapula
are winged or stick out. When the muscles in the back of the
neck shorten, the flexor muscles in the front of the neck
weaken and become overstretched.

The result is restricted or limited movement in the entire
neck and shoulder area. Headaches, abnormal muscle patterns
in the jaw such as clenching or grinding of the teeth, decreased breathing capacity, and pain in the neck and upper
back are some of the more common negative impacts of this
poor posture. In really poor posture, compression of the cervical and spinal nerves that lie deep within the lower part of
the neck occurs because the space between the clavicle (collarbone) and the first rib is decreased. This can lead to pain,
numbness, and tingling in the arms, hands, and fingers. In
extreme cases there can even be a loss of strength in the arms
or in the hands' ability to grip. If you have any of these symptoms, consult your primary health provider before beginning
these range of motion exercises or the strengthening program.

Let the Evidence Stand

I once worked with the young daughter of a local physician.
He came to me out of concern for his daughter's future health
because her posture was so bad. She was extremely tall and
willowy with a long slender neck. She had begun to slump at
a very early age, and when she came to me, she was seventeen
and already experiencing pain in her upper back. Her neck
had moved into a position several inches in front of her body,
her upper back was severely rounded, and her shoulders were
rolled in, giving her chest a hollow appearance. She couldn't
stand up straight without feeling extreme discomfort and the
range of motion in her shoulders was very restricted.

She began to work with me twice a week and did the exercises I recommended on her own every day. At the end of two months I received this letter from the physician:

We had sought several other professional opinions for her, but it was not until she started your unique exercise program that we noticed any improvement. She does the exercises daily, enjoys them, and has completely resolved her previous back problems.

His daughter was equally pleased:

I've tried so many things to improve my posture, and in a matter of weeks the exercises fixed me! I enjoyed every one of our sessions and am still keeping up with my exercises at home.

Feeling It in Your Bones

Another fairly common muscle imbalance in the neck is a condition referred to as a "military neck." It's a condition where the person has lost most or all of his cervical curve, and the neck resembles a straight rod. This often occurs following a whiplash injury. Attached to the base of the skull, the muscles in the front of the neck become constricted as a result of the whipping motion and tighten up. Because the cervical curve is created by the wedge-shaped discs, the muscles pulling the head down push onto the first vertebra and straighten out the curve in the neck. This puts increased pressure on the cervical discs, and can cause severe, chronic headaches as well as pain at the back of the head and down the back of the neck.

In the case of osteoporosis, a rounded upper back is not the result of poor posture habits. Osteoporosis is the most common disease of bones in the world. Bone loss caused by aging occurs in both men and women, the process beginning sometime after the age of forty in most individuals. Much has been written about the effects of menopause or the loss of estrogen and its effect on bones in women, but little has been written about the potentially devastating effects of this disease in men.

Men may lose from 5 to 8 percent of bone mass every ten years, starting at forty. Women lose more, between 10 and 15 percent, probably because of the hormone connection. In either case, osteoporosis can be a painful and eventually debilitating disease.

As bone density decreases, stress or crush fractures may occur, brought on by even normal daily activities. The compression of simply standing, lifting, or bending over can be enough to crush the vertebrae. This usually results in immediate, acute pain, which does subside but is often replaced by a chronic, dull ache.

These crush fractures are what are responsible for the loss in height and rounding upper back as the disease progresses. Treatment for the disease is usually bed rest and mild pain relievers following a fracture incident, and then gentle exercise to regain flexibility and muscle tone. Water exercise and walking are the exercises most often prescribed.

The exercises in this chapter are a perfect accompaniment for people with either one of these conditions. The exercises are non–weight bearing and therefore put no compression on areas already stressed. They encourage gentle movement within the joints and serve as an ideal warm-up before either swimming or walking, because they increase blood flow to the muscles and connective tissue and lubricate the joint capsules before more strenuous exercise.

Having a Good Head on Your Shoulders

There is no such thing as "perfect posture," but there is preferred posture, one that brings about skeletal alignment by the maintenance of equal tension in opposing muscles. Preferred posture allows a balanced distribution of weight and a stable position of each joint in the body (See Illustration 7).

Now realistically we know we can't force the body to completely change the habits and postural adaptations developed over a lifetime. That is not the purpose of this program. A variety of factors have created and contributed to your particular posture. The exercises and stretches in this book are designed to make measurable improvements in your body alignment and flexibility, to reduce or eliminate your pain, and to optimize your body's ability to move closer to that preferred posture.

Posture, whether good or bad, is mainly a product of habit. If we didn't care much about the way we look, maybe we would be content to continue to slouch, look shorter, and less energetic (and actually feel less energetic). Faulty posture usually causes discomfort, and then progresses to pain that often becomes chronic. That's a pretty good reason to consider correcting your posture. Even if you are reading this book and know you have poor posture but are not experiencing any pain, don't be fooled into believing that your poor posture is not affecting you.

A person can have faulty posture and still be flexible and active. If your body is not remaining in any position for long periods of time, you may not feel stiffness or pain, but continued faulty posture creates increased compression on the surfaces of your bones. If the bones are experiencing constant and repeated stresses, so are your connective tissues (tendons and ligaments). If the connective tissue is experiencing repeated stress, so are your muscles. Eventually you are going to have pain, either as a sudden onset of acute pain, which you will assume is an injury, or as an onset of moderate pain that is severe but chronic. Then you will probably attribute it to old age. If faulty posture persists you will eventually feel the effects.

In fact, the cumulative effects of constant or repeated stresses can create the same problems that sudden severe stress can. This program can start the process of reversing the effects of poor posture that you have practiced over a lifetime. You now have a tool, one that allows you to gently *persuade* the body to adapt new habits of holding and carrying itself, a program that is based on creating and maintaining balanced, well-supported, and functional strength, so that you may feel more energetic, more flexible, and better able to perform any and every task you undertake.

If you have experienced a whiplash injury and have been

released from treatment, you may begin this program. Be attentive to what you *feel* as you do each one of the moves, and remember, pain or discomfort is a signal that the exercise may not be for you or needs to be modified. If you are still under a physician or chiropractor's care, discuss this program with him or her before beginning.

If you have been diagnosed as having a military neck or have been told you have lost your cervical curve, place a small roll under your neck as you do the exercises and do not attempt to lengthen your neck toward the floor, as the instructions state. You want to maintain as much curve in your neck as you are able.

Every Little Bit Helps

This section of the book (chapters 5 through 9) is divided into four categories: range of motion exercises, strengthening exercises, moving stretches, and static or held-position stretches. Many of these moves overlap and act to stretch *and* strengthen. In some cases, an exercise will do all three—improve range of motion, stretch the body, and functionally strengthen the muscles. Each section can be done individually or may be combined to make a comprehensive program that warms and loosens up your body, strengthens all the muscles in your back, shoulders, and hips, stretches you out afterward, and completely relaxes you while you are doing all that.

Remember, this entire program is adaptable. Don't let the number of exercises included here scare you. Just as with the abdominal exercises, it is not necessary for you to do every one. Each segment has its own purpose. When done separately they produce one result; when combined in any number of ways the result will be different. Keep it simple by adjusting the program to fit your daily needs. Use the range of motion exercises only to relax and unwind at the end of one day, and then use them to loosen up in the morning.

If your schedule is flexible and you have more time on some days than others, use range of motion exercises as the warmup for the strengthening exercises two or three times a week. If your schedule is fixed and always feels too tight, break everything up into fifteen-minute segments and assign them a specific time slot in your busy day. If ten minutes is all you can spare (you certainly deserve to give yourself ten minutes!), do just one of the movements or exercises.

The more of the program you do each day, the faster you will see and feel results, but don't be overwhelmed. Doing pieces of this program is better than doing nothing at all. If you are only able to do these moves every couple of days you will still be helping your body to become more balanced by using the muscles differently from your usual pattern in your everyday activities.

The following moves are designed to guide you through various ranges of motion. They ask for movement through the full *anatomical* range of motion, but the slowness of the movement combined with your focus on what you are feeling will allow you to discover your *actual* range of motion.

The key is to stay within an area that is comfortable and above all, pain free. *If you feel any pain or impingement, or have been advised by your health care provider to avoid these positions, do not do these exercises.*

Many people have the tendency to do these range of motion exercises too quickly. Even though each move serves a very specific clinical purpose, they are meant to be done in a relaxed state that is almost meditative. You will *feel* the physical sensations associated with each movement and derive more benefit if you do them with your eyes closed. Finding your own natural rhythm, possibly by matching your slow, deep breathing with the steps in each exercise, will help make the moves fluid. Using the audio tapes offered at the back of the book will help this process.

Take it slow, and concentrate on continuous movement. By that I mean no long pauses between direction changes. You want to begin your return as soon as you have reached the end of your range of motion. When moving your arms or legs singly rather than both at once, allow the moving arm or leg to return to a completely relaxed position on the floor before beginning the move with the opposite arm or leg.

Now, go put on some soothing music, unplug the telephone, hang a DO NOT DISTURB sign on the door, and prepare to thoroughly relax and experience the sensual, luxurious nature of these moves.

The exercises that follow are meant to be done together, one right after the other. Because these exercises work progressively, you will complete all the moves on one side of your body before rolling over and repeating on the other side. These first two are the same moves you did in the abdominal strengthening section. This time your focus is on *totally* relaxing. Don't be thinking about your abdominals. They will take care of themselves.

✤ *Special Tips*
If you are in your third trimester of pregnancy, roll over onto your left side and belly-breathe in between exercises.

Exercise 22 Alternate Arm Angels in the Snow

Lie on your back with your legs extended over a pillow or roll and place your arms in the butterfly position with the palms up. *Feel* the weight of your arms and let them sink into the floor. **Slowly begin to slide one arm along the floor until it's up by your ear as the other arm slides down next to your hip** (Illustration 77). Use your breath to assist you with the timing by inhaling and exhaling deeply with each movement. Keep your arms on the floor and *keep them fully extended with the palms up throughout the movement.* Do not pause when you reach the end of your range of motion, but immediately begin to slide your arms in the opposite directions. Keep the motion going for ten or twelve slides, feeling the stretch down the side of your body and in your chest. *Do not lift your arms.* Allow them to drag on the floor as you slide them. Do not force this stretch; only go as far as feels comfortable and pain-free to your body. When you have completed the slides, return to the butterfly position and rest. **Immediately move on to the next exercise.**

Illustration 77

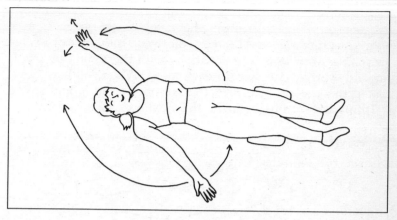

Alternate Arm Angels in the Snow

✦ *Special Tips*

If you have *any* restrictions of movement in your shoulder area, modify your arm movements to accommodate your restrictions. Do not move into an area that causes you pain or discomfort. As you continue to practice these exercises, your range of motion will increase. *Be sure not to lift your arms* during the Angels in the Snow. The friction of sliding them on the floor creates resistance that causes the muscles in the back to work, making this a strength move as well as a stretch. If you lift the arms the muscles in the chest and front of the shoulder will be working, and we want them to remain relaxed during this exercise so they may be gently stretched.

Exercise 23 Alternate Arm Sweep

Slide your right arm down next to your hip and thigh, palm down and resting on the floor. Now slide your left arm up next to the side of your head, keeping it fully extended with the palm facing up (Illustration 78). **Slowly lift both arms off the floor simultaneously and begin to exchange their positions by sweeping over the top of your body** (Illustration 79). You will be bringing your left arm down to the floor and your right arm up next to your head. Sweep them slowly back and forth, feeling the stretch down the side of your body as each arm comes up over your head. Keep the motion of your arms rhythmic and fluid as you sweep them ten or twelve times. Use your breath to assist you with the timing by inhaling and exhaling deeply with each move. When you have completed the sweeps, return to the butterfly position and rest. **Immediately move on to the next exercise.**

Illustration 78

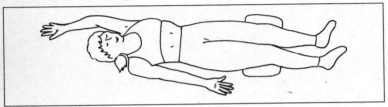

Illustration 79

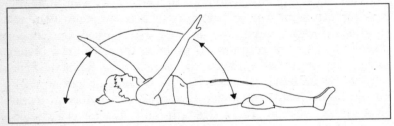

Alternate Arm Sweep

Exercise 24 Opposite Hand to Arm Move

Continuing to lie on your back with your arms outstretched, slide them down until they are level with your chest (Illustration 80). Your body will be forming a T. Lift your right arm up and slowly bring it directly across your body until your fingers touch the other arm. Don't hold the arm stiffly; let the wrist and elbow be soft (Illustration 81). Return the arm to the floor and repeat with the left arm. Keep this motion going for ten or twelve times, always returning your arm fully to the floor and relaxing it before you begin to move the other arm.

When you have completed the move with both arms, return to your starting position and rest.
Immediately move on to the next exercise.

Illustration 80

Illustration 81

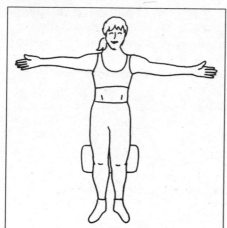 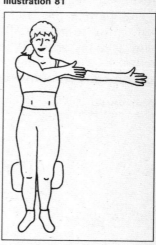

Opposite Hand to Arm Move

✤ *Special Tips*

Try to keep your arms straight, allowing them to bend only when necessary; i.e., when taking your arm across your body, let the elbow bend just as you touch your other arm. By keeping the arm in an extended position, you isolate the muscles in the back and shoulder girdle rather than using the muscles in the arms to do the move.

Exercise 25 Alternate Hand to Opposite Knee

Move your roll out from under your legs and bend your knees. Place your feet flat on the floor. Your feet and knees should be as wide apart as feels comfortable. Your arms are in a V out from your shoulders with the arms fully extended and the palms facing up (Illustration 82). With your arms, find the position that feels comfortable and doesn't strain you. **Slowly lift your right arm up and bring it diagonally** across your body. **As you reach the center of your body, roll the arm inward so that the thumb points down and touches the opposite hip bone or thigh** (Illustration 83). **Return your arm to the floor, palm up, and relax it before you begin to move the left arm.** Keep this motion going, moving the arms alternately until you have completed ten or twelve sweeps (Illustration 84). The motion should be slow and rhythmic. When you have completed the sweeps, return to your starting position and rest.

Immediately move on to the next exercise.

Illustration 82

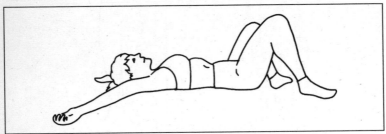

Illustration 83

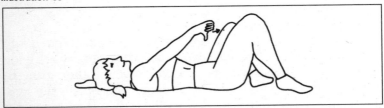

Illustration 84

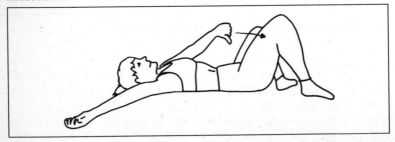

Alternate Hand to Opposite Knee

✤ *Special Tips*

In all of the above exercises, as you are moving the arms notice the difference between your right side and your left. See if you can feel which muscles are lengthening and which are shortening. Notice how the same muscles change roles from a prime mover to an assistant or stabilizer as you change directions. The same muscles that pull the arm up control the speed and stabilize the arm as it moves downward. Feel muscles moving bones, muscles stabilizing bones. Notice how a move feels like a stretch as you go in one direction, but feels more like a strength move when you reverse and go the other way.

If you feel any strain in your lower back as you move your arms over your head, pull your abdominals in and up just enough to stabilize your back without creating tension in your body.

Keep your neck and the top of your shoulders relaxed as you are doing these moves *and breathe*!

Exercise 26 Side-Lying Arm Circles

Roll over onto your right side with your head on a pillow or cradled on your bottom arm. Lift your left arm with the fingers pointed toward the ceiling and the palm facing the front of your body (Illustration 85). **Slowly begin to make a small circle with your arm, as though you were drawing small circles in a pool of water.** Keep the movement slow and rhythmic and gradually begin to increase the size of the circles (Illustration 86). Concentrate on *feeling* the movement of the arm in the shoulder joint. Notice any restriction or discomfort within the circles and keep the motion within a range that is free from pain. Enlarge the circle as big as is comfortable for your body (Illustration 87). (Your goal is for the arm to be circling close to your hip, your chest, your head, and as far back as feels comfortable.) Now reverse the motion and go the other direction. Gradually decrease the size of the circles until your fingers are once again pointed toward the ceiling.

Immediately move on to the next exercise.

Illustration 85

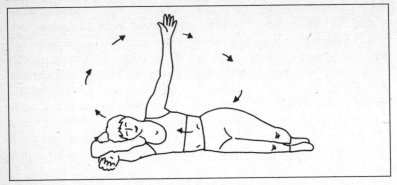

Side-Lying Arm Circles.

Illustration 86

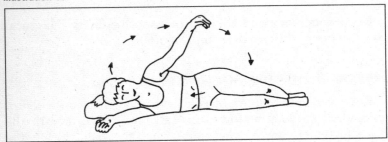

Small circles with arm. Enlarge slowly to big circles.

Illustration 87

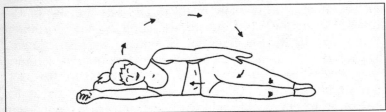

Reverse direction and slowly return to small circles.

Exercise 27 Side-Lying Elbow Circles

In the same position, bend your arm, letting it hang free, and point your elbow at the ceiling (Illustration 88). **Begin to make small circles with your elbow, concentrating on feeling the movement of the entire shoulder girdle as you move.** Circle slowly, gradually increasing the size of the circles until your arm is close to your hip, your chest, your head, and as far back as feels comfortable (Illustration 89). Feel the movement of the shoulder blade against your back, moving up, back, down, and forward. **When the circles are as large as your body allows them to be** (Illustration 90), **reverse and go in the opposite direction, beginning large and gradually decreasing the circumference of the cir-**

Illustration 88

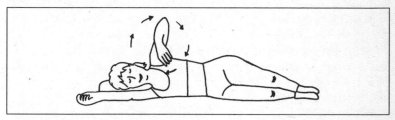

Illustration 89

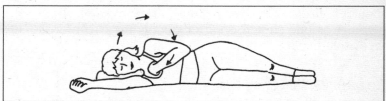

Illustration 90

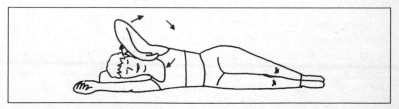

Side-Lying Elbow Circles

cles until your elbow is once again pointed toward the ceiling. Feel your range of motion and notice any restriction or tightness as you move both directions. Stay within a range that is comfortable and pain-free.
Immediately move on to the next exercise.

❖ *Special Tips*
Make sure you remain lying on your side and without allowing your body to roll forward or backward as you circle your arm. Allow the natural rotation of the hand and arm as you circle it.

Once again, pay very close attention to what you are feeling. *Any* discomfort or pain is a signal that you are moving more than your body is ready to. Feeling the tension from the stretch is okay. It may feel a little uncomfortable at first. So will using muscles you are not accustomed to using.

Make the circles *slowly*. Most people move too quickly, not giving the joint capsule time to lubricate. Exercises 22 through 25 help prepare the shoulder area for the circular movement, but ligaments (they connect bone to bone) do not have the blood supply available that muscles do; therefore they take longer to warm up.

Exercises 28 and 29 are also in the moving stretch section of the book, but because they improve range of motion in the shoulder girdle, they are included here as well. They work together as one stretch, so after completing this exercise, immediately begin the next.

Exercise 28 Side-Lying Arm Slide

Still lying on your side, extend your arms in front of you on the floor. They should be at chest level with your palms touching each other (Illustration 91). **Slowly slide your top arm forward, letting it rest on the floor, and let your head and neck roll forward naturally** (Illustration 92). When you have gone as far as your arm can go, **slide it up about 45 degrees toward your head.** Keep the palm on the floor (Illustration 93). Only go as far as is comfortable and feel the stretch down the side of your back. **Slide your hand**

**back down until your palms are touching and then slide
your arm backward, keeping it straight and allowing your
shoulder blade to move** (Illustration 94). Do not let your
body roll back as the arm slides. You want to isolate the movement in the shoulder blade. Repeat the sequence slides several
times, then come back to your starting position and rest.

Immediately move on to the next exercise.

Illustration 91

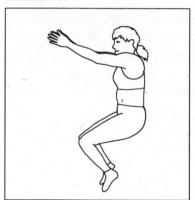

Illustration 92

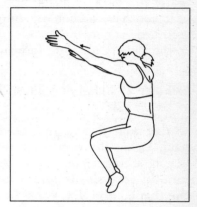

Illustration 93

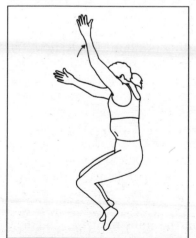

Illustration 94

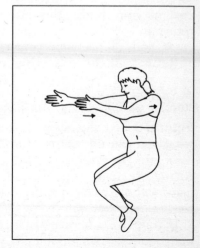

Side-Lying Arm Slide

✤ *Special Tips*
The first slide will be a little stiff, but as you continue the movement you will feel the shoulder blade sliding forward and backward as you slide your arm. The trick is not to bend your arm. Keeping the arm straight forces the move to come from the shoulder girdle, and that's what you want.

As with Angels in the Snow, be careful not to lift the arm off the floor. In this case, the friction will enhance the stretching of the muscles in the upper and middle back.

If you have a shoulder impingement and movement over your head is not comfortable, do not do the 45-degree portion of the slide. Only slide forward and backward.

Exercise 29 Side-Lying Chest Stretch

While still on your side, lift your left arm up and extend it so that your fingers are pointed toward the ceiling with the palm facing the front of your body (Illustration 95). Inhale deeply through your nose. **As you exhale through your mouth, very slowly allow your extended arm to lower to the back, and let your head, neck, and chest follow.** When your arm has gone as far as your muscles will allow it to go comfortably, **release into the stretch and relax the rest of your body** (Illustration 96). When you are ready to return to your side, bend your elbow, place your hand on your chest, and roll back into your resting position (Illustration 97). **Repeat all the side-lying exercises on the other side.**

✤ *Special Tips*
This stretch may be very difficult for someone with very forward rolled shoulders. Listen to your body. Let it dictate what you can do. Letting the arm back very slowly will help ease into the stretch. If you cannot touch the floor without rolling over onto your back, it's okay to roll over. *Make sure you bend your elbow and place your hand on your chest before rolling back onto your side.*

If you have a herniated disc in the lumbar region, this may not be safe or comfortable for you to do. *If you know twisting motions cause you discomfort, do not do this stretch.* In any

Illustration 95

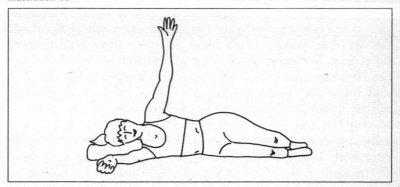

Illustration 96   **Illustration 97**

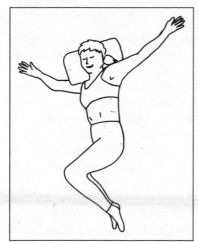 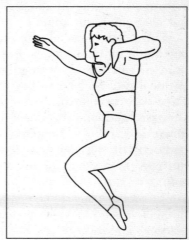

Side-Lying Chest Stretch

event, move slowly and *feel* how your lower back responds rather than just rolling into it.

As you are doing the program regularly, notice how your range of motion increases as you continue to do each of these moves. The increase may be very small at first, but by repeating the exercises every day, your flexibility will continue to improve.

Remember, your muscles pull your bones closer together, so even after stretching, muscles that are overly tight can actually pull your body back into its original position. You'll eliminate this recoil response, which often happens after static or held stretching, by doing these range of motion exercises and the moving stretches. The recoil response is greatly reduced by the slow release or sneaking out theory applied to the strengthening exercises and sustained stretches in this program.

As it was mentioned earlier, use these exercises in as many ways as you can imagine. You may do them as a way to loosen your body up first thing in the morning, as a way to unwind at the end of the day, or as a prelude to the strengthening exercises that follow in the next chapter. I often do them as a form of moving meditation that not only relaxes my body but also quiets my mind.

If you have special circumstances that prevent you from beginning more strenuous exercise at this time, or you simply want to ease into a strengthening program, these moves are an ideal way for you to begin a gentle strengthening regime. They are wonderful for seniors and anyone with limited strength, and may be done in a firm bed if you cannot get down on the floor. Remember, the secret is to listen to your body. Let it tell you what it is able and willing to do. All of the movements may be adapted to your range of motion. *Be willing to start small and allow your body to increase its ability to move when it is ready.* However you choose to use them, I hope you allow yourself to become immersed in the physical sensation of the movement and total relaxation.

6

Getting to the Bottom
of Things

We've talked about the upper body; now let's talk about the lower half, the center of gravity and the places where gravity often takes its biggest toll!

It is almost impossible to have correctly aligned posture in the upper body and poor posture in the lower half. Our bodies work as wholly integrated units. And when poor posture extends to the lumbar spine, two situations commonly occur.

If you have excessive curvature in your lower back, the muscles directly over that area will be shortened and may become overly tight, as will the hip flexors and the muscles down the outside of the hip and thigh. The opposing muscle groups, primarily the abdominals and the gluteus maximus (buttocks) tend to further weaken, which contributes to an already unstable posture.

I also commonly see people with flat back syndrome, or a loss of the lumbar curve. It's one of the things that happen when the hamstrings and hips become overly tightened and pull the spine into a slightly flexed position, keeping the muscles in the lower back continuously lengthened. In this case, the hip flexors (the opposing muscle group) become overstretched and weak. The most superficial abdominal muscle, the rectus abdominis, is usually overly shortened from being held in a flexed position. The shortened rectus abdominis pulls the rib cage down and creates the appearance of a sunken, hollow chest. This combination leads to overstretched and weakened spinal ligaments, and the result is instability of the pelvis and lumbar spine.

In both these scenarios, the individual is likely to suffer from chronic back pain. Because of the altered biomechanics of movement caused by the postural imbalances, all the adjacent muscles and connective tissue are under constant stress. The range of motion and strengthening exercises in this chapter concentrate on the lower body. They encourage full range of motion in the lumbar spine, in the pelvis, and in the hips, helping to restore balance and increase stability, flexibility, and strength.

The *pelvis* (from the Latin word meaning *basin*) is made up of several bones supported by the largest muscles in the body. Each side of the pelvis has three parts, and the junction of these three bony parts forms the hip socket. The head of the femur (the thigh bone) sits in this socket. These three elements that make up the bony pelvis are separate parts in the developing fetus and in an infant but they become fused together by adulthood, very much like the bones of the skull.

Although it is difficult to see where these separate bones join, they are nevertheless referred to by three separate names: the *ilium, ischium,* and the *os pubis.* The ilia are wing shaped and form the top half of the pelvis. Many major muscles are attached to these smooth, curvaceous bones we call our hip bones, including the abdominal muscles, the gluteus maximus, the latissimus dorsi (sometimes called "lats"), and the outer muscles of the thigh.

The bottom of the pelvis is composed of the ischium and the os pubis. The ischium forms the back of the pelvis and is the attachment for the large muscles in the back of the leg, the hamstrings, and the muscles on the inside of the thigh. These muscles play a key role in a balanced posture. The os pubis is at the front and bottom of the pelvis and serves as the lowest attachment for muscles in the abdomen.

The hip bones are connected to a third bone called the *sacrum.* The sacrum is a wedge-shaped, concave bone that is smooth on its front surface, and rough and bumpy on the back, where several muscles and ligaments attach. Like the hip bones, the sacrum is also made up of bones—five fused vertebrae—that form a wedge. At the junctions where the vertebrae meet, small openings are formed, through which the sacral nerves exit.

The top of the sacrum joins the last lumbar vertebra, L5, and the bottom joins the *coccyx* or tailbone. The sacrum is connected to the pelvis and to the lumbar vertebrae by a network of thick, strong ligaments. These ligaments are the strongest in the body, and adjust their tension according to body movement. (The weight of the body forces the sacrum downward between the hip bones, exerting a pull that causes the ligaments to hold more firmly. This pull or pressure is what stabilizes the pelvis.)

Ligaments are thick bundles of parallel fibers that are mainly composed of collagenous material; therefore ligaments are very strong but not very elastic. Their primary function is to check excessive motion and stabilize the joint. They do not contract the way muscle tissue does, nor do they actively stretch. They have a mildly elastic component that comes from the spiral orientation of their fibers. Ligaments contain many sensory nerve cells that constantly transmit information to the brain about the speed, movement, and position of the joint. The brain then sends signals to the muscles to slow down, shift position, or in some other way alter the movement to avoid stress and damage to the ligaments.

The ligaments that hold the head of the femur in the joint capsule are not only strong, but their spiral component also plays a large role in the range of motion. Rotating the leg inward increases their spiral, so movement in this direction tends to be limited. External or outward rotation unwinds the spiral fibers. When flexion and external rotation are combined, the ligaments are all relaxed, as when you are sitting with your knees wide apart. Movement of the joint is controlled by the muscles surrounding it. As strong as the ligaments are, they are still susceptible to sprain or rupture if movement is excessive or the joint experiences trauma.

Movements of the pelvis involve simultaneous movement of the lumbar spine and the hip joint. When the pelvis is rotated forward or upward, it flattens out the curve in the lumbar spine. This can act as a mild stretch. As the pelvis moves backward or downward and tilts back, there is an increase in the curve. Tilting up one side of the pelvis creates a lateral (side) bending of the spine. All these actions are necessary for functional movement.

The hip is a ball-and-socket joint, allowing movement in all directions. Restrictions of motion in the hip joint affect all the nearby structures, namely the lower back and the knees. Hips (like shoulders) are very individual. For instance, there is a significant difference between the male and female pelvis. Females have a wider pelvis and the orientation of the bones is different to provide for childbearing. Pelvises come in all sizes and shapes. Some are wider, some are longer. Some are more curved than others. These differences all affect the position of the hip socket, and therefore the range of motion of a particular individual.

The elasticity of connective tissue also varies from one person to another and is affected by a variety of factors. Scar tissue that results from any trauma to the joint will lessen the elasticity of the ligaments. Connective tissue is 70 percent water, so being well hydrated is essential for the health and pliability of the tissues. In other words, each person's experience with movement is going to be different.

The Seat of the Trouble

The gluteus maximus is the largest muscle in the body, and together with layers of body fat, is what shapes our rear end. The primary action of the gluteus maximus is to extend or pull the thigh backward. It is a prime mover in straightening up from a bent-over position, walking up stairs, and any other movement that requires powerful extension of the leg. When standing, the direction of the gluteal contraction is reversed, and this muscle assists in holding the pelvis in correct alignment under the rib cage. In other words, it pulls the buttocks toward the leg rather than pulling the leg backward as it does in walking. It is a major stabilizer of the hip joint and even affects the stability of the knees when we're walking and standing.

The gluteus maximus is another muscle that has been affected by the change in our daily activities. As I just described, the "gluts" are working whenever we are standing or moving. Unfortunately, most of our daily activities involve sitting. Sitting puts this large muscle on *stretch,* and sitting for long periods of time leads to an *overstretched,* weakened muscle. This same sitting position contributes to short, tight hamstrings, which play a huge role in lower back pain. We'll talk more about that in the next chapter.

Sciatica, or pain that radiates from the buttock down the leg, is a common complaint. Sometimes the pain starts in the lower back; often it does not. It may even travel down into the foot and be accompanied by numbness or tingling. The pain indicates that there is pressure being put on the sciatic nerve that lies deep in the buttock. If someone has a herniated or bulging disc, or even severe disc degeneration, the disc material may push out and press upon the sciatic nerve at the junction of the last vertebra, L-5, and the sacrum. This can cause intense pain and should be treated by a professional health care provider.

If there has been no history of injury that would suggest a herniated disc, and particularly if there is no lower back pain, there can be another source of the pressure on the nerve. That brings us to another muscle, the *piriformis.* The piriformis lies underneath the gluteus maximus and directly *across* the opening in the pelvis where the sciatic nerve exits and extends down.

The common assumption has been that an overly tight piriformis was the culprit. Appropriate stretching exercises are thought to alleviate the problem. But occasionally the problem is a *flaccid* or overly weak piriformis muscle. When the piriformis muscle has normal or good tone, it bridges over the sciatic nerve, allowing the nerve to exit into the leg without contact. When it is overstretched or weak, it flattens out and can put direct pressure on the nerve.

The piriformis muscle is an external rotator of the hip and leg. People who have feet and legs that are extremely turned out (duck-footed) are likely to have an overly contracted piriformis muscle. People who have a tendency to turn their toes in, or sit with their legs crossed a lot, are more likely to have a weakened, overstretched muscle. If you suffer from sciatica, pay attention to whether any of the positions in the following exercises bring on or increase sciatic pain. If so, refrain from those movements.

This chapter has exercises for improving range of motion *and* for strengthening the lower body. The range of motion exercises will act as a warm-up for the strengthening exercises that follow. You will finish up with more range of motion moves that act as gentle stretches before you go on to the back exercises.

The Bicycle Pump exercise that follows puts the hip and knee joints through all their functional and anatomical ranges of motion. It serves to warm up the lower body before exercise or to gently loosen up the body before beginning the day's activities. It acts as a mild stretch for the large muscle groups and prepares the lower back for movement. It prepares the hips and lower back for the knee rolls to come.

Exercise 30 Bicycle Pump with External Rotation

Lie on your side with your knees bent and together. Pull your top leg up to your chest and then begin to open the leg out and downward as if you were riding a bicycle (Illustrations 98 and 99). As the leg extends down and straightens out, sweep it back, stretching the front of the body and feeling the contraction in your buttock (Illustration 100). With your leg held back, bend your knee to stretch the front of the thigh (Illustration 101). Pull knee back up to the starting position, then open top leg out to the side, keeping knee bent (Illustration 102). Do not allow your body to roll with the leg. Return your bent knee to starting position and repeat sequence six times.

Repeat on other side.

✤ *Special Tips*
If you have had a hip replacement, ask your primary health care practitioner if it is safe for you to practice this exercise. The following cue words may help you remember the sequence of movements:

Illustration 98

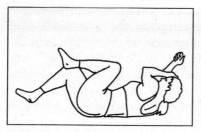

Illustration 99

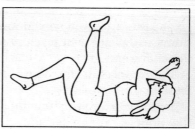

Illustration 100

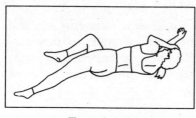

Illustration 101

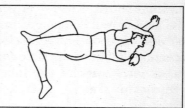

Illustration 102

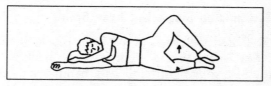

Bicycle Pump with External Rotation

Pull up	Pull up to other knee
Open out	Open up
Sweep back	Return to starting position
Bend knee	

Keep the hand of your top arm on the floor to prevent your body from rolling forward or backward as you go through the moves.

The next exercises strengthen the hips, buttocks, and thighs, which play important roles in a strong and healthy back. Now here's a fun surprise: These exercises are not only good

strengtheners for the buttocks, they are incredible shapers and
sculptors. And don't pretend you aren't interested in having a
great butt. You men should know from all the advertising that
this is one of the first places women look when they're "checking out" a guy. I've been teaching these exercises in my Body
Sculpture classes for years and have seen the results for
myself!

The first exercise strengthens the gluteus medius, which is
the muscle on the outside of the upper hip, and a primary
stabilizer of the pelvis. You will probably not feel it in your
hip, but you will feel it in your thigh. Although it does work
the legs as well, keeping your pelvis level is strengthening the
outside of your hip. It will also improve your balance immensely. Pulling your abdominals in and up and keeping your
pelvis level are the key things to remember. (This is *great*
exercise for skiers!)

Exercise 31 Standing Single-Leg Knee Bend

On a raised, flat surface such as a stair or block, stand on your
right foot. Keep your body weight over the back half of your
foot. Lightly rest your right hand on a bannister or chair back
for balance and flex your left foot (Illustration 103). Do not
allow your toe to drop down (Illustration 104). **Pull your
abdominals in and up** and contract your buttocks *without*
tilting your pelvis forward. Lengthen your spine and relax the
top of your shoulders and neck, looking straight ahead, not
down at your feet. **Keeping your hips absolutely level,
slowly bend your right knee and lower your left foot
about 3 or 4 inches** (Illustration 105). If your balance is
shaky only lower yourself 2 inches. *The goal is to keep your
hips level,* not to see how far down you are able to go. As
your strength increases you will be able to go lower. Allow
your left foot to barely touch the floor, keeping all of your
weight on your right foot. Slowly press back up, pushing off
the bottom of your right foot. Use the muscles in your thigh
to raise you, keeping your body weight over the back half of
your foot.

Repeat 6 times, then change to the other leg. Do 2 sets on each leg, resting in between.

Illustration 103   Illustration 104   Illustration 105

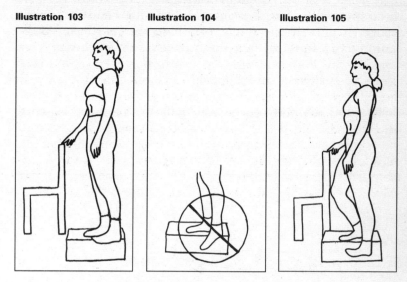

Standing Single-Leg Knee Bend

❖ *Special Tips*

This exercise requires a lot of concentration. You need to pay attention to several things at one time—back straight, shoulders relaxed, hips level, weight on back of foot, abdominals in. It is a powerful exercise for the hips and thighs if done correctly. Done incorrectly, such as with your body weight too far forward, can put stress on your knees. It is helpful if it can be done in front of a mirror. That way you may see your posture and visually check the levelness of your hips. Doing the exercise slowly increases its effectiveness.

Exercise 32 Prone Gluteal Squeeze Lift

On the floor, lie on your stomach with your forehead resting on the backs of your hands. Your legs should be spread about 12 inches apart with your toes pointed out and down (similar to a ballet position 2). Pull your abdominals **in and up** but keep your buttocks completely relaxed. **Now, squeeze the buttocks together tightly** (Illustration 106). **Slowly lift your extended legs off the floor and hold** (Illustration 107). Do not raise higher than 2 inches from the floor and don't allow your legs to bend at the knee. *Do not arch your back.* **Maintaining the squeeze in your buttocks, slowly lower your legs to the floor.** Release the contraction in your buttocks. Keep your abdominals in and up and relax the rest of your body.

    Eight repetitions equal one set; Do two sets, resting in between.

Illustration 106

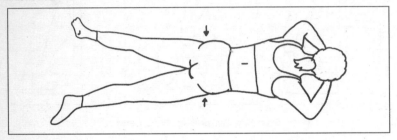

Illustration 107

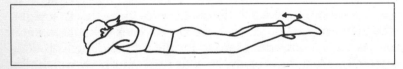

Prone Gluteal Squeeze Lift

❖ *Special Tips*
    Although you will feel the muscles in your lower back working, they are working to stabilize only. They should not be doing any of the lifting. Keeping your abdominals pulled in and up *throughout* the exercise is crucial. The internal obliques will hold the pelvis firmly in place and prevent you from hyperextending your back as you lift. *Do not lift too high.* This is the most common mistake. A very small lift (1 or 2 inches)

is all that's necessary. The smaller you make the lift, the more effectively you will isolate the muscles in your buttocks. Lifting more than the 1 or 2 inches will automatically involve the muscles in the lower back and you don't want that. Keeping your legs straight while you do the lift is also important. Again, our goal is to isolate the muscles in the buttocks. If you allow your knees to bend as you lift, you will be using the muscles in the back of your thighs, the hamstrings. If you happen to have tight hamstrings and cannot fully straighten your legs, simply hold them still as you lift and don't allow your knees to bend any further. *If this exercise bothers your lower back when you follow the instructions carefully, simply squeeze the buttocks and do not lift your legs.*

Exercise 33 Bridges

Lie on your back with your knees bent, your feet about 4 inches apart. Angle your arms down in a **V**, palms down (Illustration 108). **Pull your abdominals in and up and contract your buttocks as you lift your body so that you're resting on the back of your shoulders** (Illustration 109). Lift your body as a unit, keeping your rib cage and pelvis level. Do not lead with your pelvis; this is not a pelvic tilt (Illustration 110). Slowly lower your body until you make contact with the floor, then immediately lift again. Keep your buttocks contracted tightly throughout the move and lift and lower slowly, eight times. Return to starting position and rest.

Eight repetitions equal one set; do two or three sets. Follow with Double Bent Knee Body Curl Stretch.

✤ *Special Tips*

A good way to ensure you are lifting your body up as a unit is to *envision* half a glass of water on your abdomen. Lift your body as though it were one piece, making sure you don't spill a drop of water from the glass. Now even though I am telling you to lift carefully, *don't do this exercise too slowly*. The lifting and lowering of your body should be rhythmic and continuous. In other words, do not pause in between lowering your pelvis and the next lift. Keep it smooth. This exercise

Illustration 108

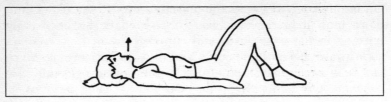

Illustration 109

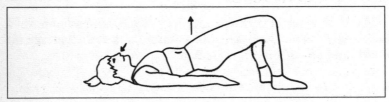

Illustration 110

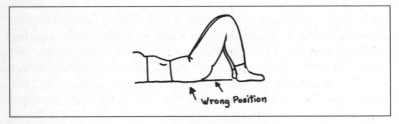

Wrong Position

Bridges

really works the hamstrings as well as the buttocks. *If your hamstrings are already too tight, this may not be an appropriate exercise for you.* If you do the exercise, make sure you properly stretch your hamstrings afterwards. (See chapter 8.)

The next two exercises are done standing or sitting rather than lying down. They are *very* effective strengtheners for the gluteals and several other muscle groups. Don't be intimidated by the squats; they are easier to do than you think, once you get the hang of them. *But,* they are hard work and will make your heart beat a little faster as well as fatigue your thighs. Take it easy at first. Don't try to do too many of them or do them too fast. When you feel your legs start to burn, sit down and immediately begin the gluteal squeezes. If you feel a little off-balance at first, place the bench or chair next to a table or counter that you can use for support.

Caution: *If you have any type of heart condition or have had knee replacement, check with your primary health care provider before attempting the squats.*

Exercise 34 Bench Squats

Stand in front of a bench or chair that is approximately 14 inches high. Your back is to the bench and your feet should be about hip-width apart. Your arms are close to your body with your palms touching the fronts of your thighs (Illustration 111). **Pulling your abdominals in and up to support your back, contract your buttocks tightly and slowly lower your backside as though you were going to sit on the bench.** Raise your arms to chest level as you lower your body. Squat until the backs of your thighs lightly touch the bench (Illustration 112), then slowly push back up to a full standing position, keeping your buttocks contracted throughout the move. *Do not allow your body weight to rest on the bench.*

Continue the squat move for 2 sets of 12 repetitions each, focusing on doing the move slowly and with tension in the gluteal muscles. On the last repetition, lower your body weight down even slower and immediately begin the next exercise.

✤ *Special Tips*
We all sit down many times a day and never think about it. Yet as soon as I tell people to "sit back as though you were sitting down" they can't seem to do it. You have to reach back with your rear end when you sit down, so remember to stick out your butt. The movement in this exercise is no different. There's a tendency to tuck the butt under, which renders the exercise ineffective. Remember, the lengthening contraction is the one that makes the muscle strong. Sticking your rear end out *stretches* the muscle fibers. Standing up shortens them. You achieve that lengthening contraction by keeping

Illustration 111   **Illustration 112**

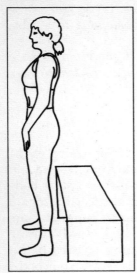 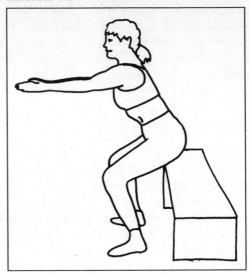

Bench Squats

tension in them, *squeezing* your cheeks as you sit back and as
you stand up. It's not easy, but I wouldn't ask you to do
something that was impossible. Don't worry about the position
of your arms. Do whatever helps you balance.

Exercise 35 Seated Gluteal Squeezes

Sit on a bench or flat-bottomed chair with your feet together flat on the floor. Make sure your hips are a little higher
than the top of your thighs and your feet are directly under
your knees (Illustrations 113 and 114). Sit with your back erect
and your abdominals pulled **in and up.** Rhythmically contract
and release your gluteal muscles (buttocks). Squeeze your
cheeks as tightly as you can, concentrating on tightening the
muscles in the lower abdomen and pelvic floor (Illustrations
115 and 116). *Do not allow your lower back to round.* Sit tall
on the bench.

Contract 12 to 16 times, then contract and hold. Hold for

Illustration 113

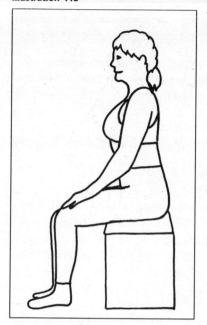

Illustration 114

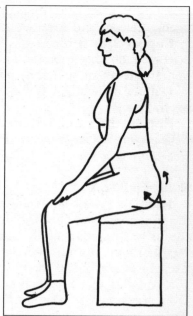

Illustration 115

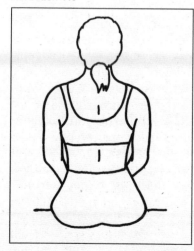

Illustration 116

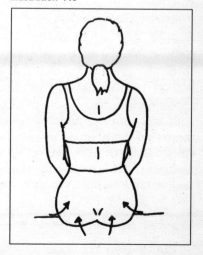

Seated Gluteal Squeezes

a slow count of ten, keeping your neck, chest, and shoulders relaxed. Release and immediately contract 12 to 16 times again. Release and rest.

Repeat 2 or 3 times.

If you do this exercise following the bench squats, after your third set of squeezes, push back up onto your feet and repeat the bench squats for another 2 sets of 12 repetitions each.

Repeat the combination 3 times.

These are all large-muscle exercises and should not be done two days in a row.

❖ *Special Tips*

Here, too, the lengthening contraction is what you're after. By squeezing your cheeks tightly while you are sitting, you are intensely strengthening the gluteals. Because you are sitting on top of them, you are literally lifting weight. Your own! This exercise is also one of the best things you can do to strengthen the muscles of reproduction and elimination. If you suffer from incontinence, this exercise can make a real difference. This is one of the exercises that prompted the letter from the couple about the improvement in their married sex life!

Now let's finish with a few more range of motion exercises to relax and gently stretch your hips. You will be using your breath consciously throughout these exercises, inhaling deeply through your nose and exhaling slowly through your mouth. Allow the rhythm of your breathing to help you time your movements.

If you have a herniated disc in the lumbar region, this next move may not be safe or comfortable for you to do. *If you know twisting motions cause you discomfort do not do this next move.* If you do this moving stretch, move slowly and *feel* how your low back responds rather than just rolling into it.

Exercise 36 Double Bent-Knee Rolls

Lie on your back, bend your knees, and place your feet and knees together. Your arms should be in the butterfly stretch, palms up. **Slowly let your knees roll to the right** (Illustration 117). (Don't *put* your knees to the right; go only as far as your muscles will let you go.) Return to the starting position, then roll your knees to the left. This is a passive move, not an active one. Allow your breath to assist you by exhaling as your knees roll to the side and inhaling as you return to center. After about ten knee rolls from side to side, add the head movement: **rotate in the *opposite* direction from your knees** (Illustration 118). After about ten rolls, add arm movement: **As you roll your knees left and head right, rotate your right palm down so that it touches the floor** (Illustration 119). *The rotation should be from the shoulder, not the wrist.* Reverse. Breathing deeply, continue to slowly roll and rotate the body until you feel your range of motion increasing and your body loosening up.

Illustration 117   **Illustration 118**   **Illustration 119**

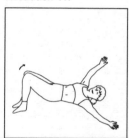 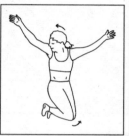 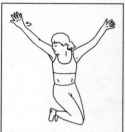

Double Bent-Knee Rolls

✤ *Special Tips*

The key to this move is to think of it as passive rather than active. Even though you are in conscious control of your movement, let gravity and the weight of your legs actually pull your knees to the side. It is also important to keep moving from one side to the other. Resist the tendency to pause when you get to each side. Since the purpose of this move is increased joint mobility, allow the muscles to get their stretch from the *movement,* not from holding the stretched position.

As with the Side-Lying Chest Stretch, if you have a compromised disc in the lumbar region, this may not be an appropriate move for you. Try the move very gently at first, and keep your range of motion small. At the first sign of discomfort, reduce the size of your movement to stay within a range that is comfortable. If even small rotation of the knees causes pain in your lower back, discontinue the exercise. After you have been doing the abdominal exercise program for a longer time, and begin to feel increased strength and stability in your lower back, you may try the exercise again.

Exercise 37 Supine Pelvic Pump

Lie on your back with your knees bent, your feet about 12 inches apart (Illustration 120). **Gently contract your buttocks and curl your pelvis up toward the ceiling,** feeling

Illustration 120

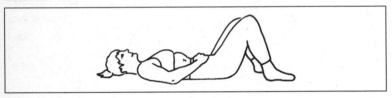

Illustration 121

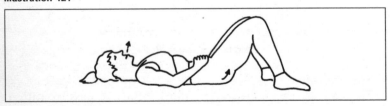

Illustration 122

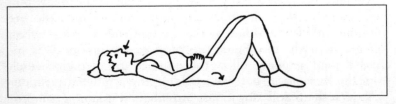

Supine Pelvic Pump

the lower back stretch as it presses into the floor (Illustration 121). **Then slowly tilt the hips down into the floor, feeling the lower back move slightly away from the floor** (Illustration 122). DO NOT ARCH YOUR BACK! Once again, use your breath throughout the move. Exhale each time you curl up, inhale each time you rotate down. Tilt your hips back and forth in slow, continuous motion for four to six pumps. Return to neutral and completely relax.

Exercise 38 Single-Knee Roll-ins

Caution: If you have had a hip replacement, do not attempt this next exercise.

Still lying on your back, with knees bent, move your feet and knees apart as wide as they can comfortably go (Illustration 123). Hold your knees straight and don't let them roll

Illustration 123

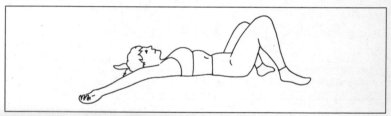

out to the sides. **Slowly rotate the left knee in while the right knee stays up** (Illustration 124). Return to starting position and repeat with the other knee. (Don't press your knee in, allow the muscles to control how far you rotate.) Breathing deeply, exhale on each roll-in and inhale as you return your knee to center. Keep repeating the single-knee roll-ins about ten times, then add arm movement: rotate the palm of your right hand toward the floor as your right knee rolls in (Illustration 125). Again, rotate from the shoulder, not the wrist. Last, add head movement: as you roll your right knee in and right palm down, rotate your head to the left (Illustration 126). Continue to roll slowly and rotate until you feel your range of motion increasing and your body loosening up.

Illustration 124

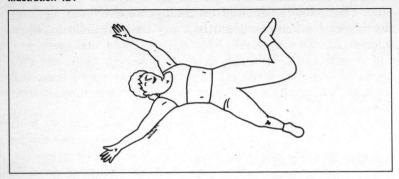

Illustration 125

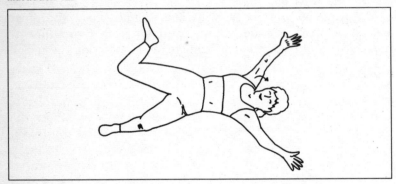

Illustration 126

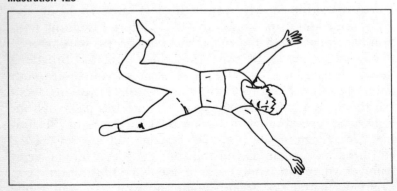

Single-Knee Roll-ins

This first stretch will be repeated in chapter 7, but it is a great one and you can do it several times during your workout if you enjoy it. Read the instructions carefully before beginning. *Don't skip any steps.*

Exercise 39 Double Bent-Knee Body Curl

Lie on your back with your knees bent. Lift your feet off the floor and bring your knees up into a 90-degree angle, holding the outside of your knees with your hands. Allow the legs to open wide to stretch the buttocks (Illustration 127). Find "neutral" with your lower back and rest there. Inhale deeply through your nose, and as you exhale, **slowly pull your knees into your chest and gently lift your hips off the floor,** keeping the knees apart (Illustration 128). Feel the stretch in your lower back area. Inhale deeply, and as you exhale, **slowly tuck your chin and curl your upper body up toward your knees** (Illustration 129). Feel the stretch in your upper and middle back. Gentle lower your upper body, keeping your knees pulled to your chest. *Stop and allow the back to relax.* Slowly lower the hips to the floor, but keep hold of your knees. Find "neutral" with your back. Slowly lower your feet to the floor and allow your back to relax. Extend your legs out over your rolled towel or pillow. Completely relax and belly-breathe.

Repeat 1 time.

Illustration 127   **Illustration 128**   **Illustration 129**

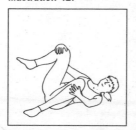
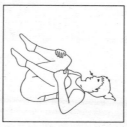
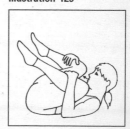

Double Bent-Knee Body Curl

By now you should be as loose as a noodle, completely relaxed, and ready for whatever the day may bring. If you did these range of motion exercises as a prelude to the strengthening program, then move on to the next chapter.

If you have done all you are going to for today, prolong the experience by staying in a state of body awareness all day. Stay "tuned in" to the physical sensations you feel as you go about your daily activities. Notice where and when you feel tension accumulating in any of your muscles.

Notice where and when you feel fatigue or discomfort in any part of your body. Notice if you feel a little looser, less stiff. In *Ageless Body, Timeless Mind*, Deepak Chopra says: "To have a renewed body, you must be willing to have new perceptions that give rise to new solutions." So pay attention to yourself.

These range of motion exercises can give you a new perception of your own flexibility. You'll learn that you have the ability to move in ways you never thought possible. That knowledge can open up a vast new universe to you—one that involves unrestricted, uninhibited movement.

At the Monterey Bay Aquarium in Monterey, my favorite marine animals are the Moon Jellies. These ancient, translucent creatures move without thought. Their movements are continuous, mesmerizing, and hauntingly beautiful—graceful and fluid motions by bodies that have no bones.

As you do these exercises, imagine that you have no bones. Let yourself feel as free floating as a Moon Jelly. Get to know yourself in a whole new way.

PART III

Back-Strengthening Program

7

Back to Back Basics

I hate to pull you out of the wonderful, relaxed place you are in, but if you've just completed the exercises in the last chapter, we need to get on with the business of strengthening. In the exercises in the previous chapters, relaxation has played a very important role. In this chapter the focus will be on muscle tension. We'll use principles similar to those described in the abdominal exercises: exaggerating the positions of the body, holding contractions in the muscles involved for a slow count, and then a slow release followed by relaxation. The main difference is the number of muscles involved.

Each exercise will involve the muscles in your neck, spine, shoulder girdle, chest, buttocks, and, of course, your abdominals. Most of the exercises are strengthening the muscles in one area of your body, while sustaining a gentle stretch in the opposing muscle group. Every muscle in your back and shoulder girdle will be strengthened with this program. You'll isolate specific muscles with careful positioning of your arms.

The purpose of exaggerated positions is to create new muscle memory. Holding your body in these positions for several seconds sends a message to the central nervous system that will be retained deep in your brain. This message is repeated each time you do the exercise. Soon your muscles will assume a modified version of these exercises in your everyday posture and movement.

Straight from the Shoulder

Your shoulder blades (scapula) are suspended over your rib cage by a network of muscles and ligaments. They literally hang on your back. Because they "float" rather than being fixed in position, they can move in many directions. The ability of the scapula to move freely determines the range of movement of the arms. A person who has a frozen shoulder, impingement syndrome, or a rotator cuff injury usually has restricted motion of the arm. Movements of the arms involve the muscles in the midback, chest, and rib cage. Therefore someone who has an injury that limits arm and shoulder movement will also have reduced or impaired strength in his or her back muscles. Protecting the injured shoulder with cautious arm movements prevents full functional use of the back muscles.

The muscles in the shoulder girdle switch roles and the direction of their contraction depending on what they are called upon to do. Several muscles are considered both muscles of the spine and also of the shoulder girdle. Many play a key role in respiration. For instance, the pectoralis minor is a postural muscle deep in the chest that is attached to the front of the shoulder blade and to the rib cage. It pulls the scapula forward and downward, and is usually involved in the hunched-forward shoulder posture that results from prolonged sitting with arms in a forward position—e.g., driving or typing. It also assists in respiration, helping to lift the ribs during inhalation. In both cases it brings bones closer together, but it reverses the direction of its contracting to perform the secondary task.

The function of the trapezius is another example of how muscles can change roles. The trapezius assists in movement of the midback and shoulder girdle.

This large, diamond-shaped muscle has three distinct sets of fibers that can work together to perform a task, or separately to perform independent actions. In the neck, the upper fibers of the trapezius extend the neck backward and also rotate and flex the head to the side. In the midback, all of its fibers contract at once to pull the scapula together. This action opens the chest and front of the shoulder area, and is necessary to achieve postural alignment. Its lower fibers pulls the scapula downward to stabilize it against the rib cage and assist in upward rotation when the arm is lifted forward. It also plays a role in extension of the spine.

A muscle may be strong in one capacity but ineffective in another. It may be adaptively shortened but weak. When a muscle is held in a shortened position, the fibers cannot contract any further. The muscle may be holding the bones closer to each other firmly, but by definition it isn't strong if it cannot contract. Strength comes from the elastic ability of muscle to pull, not just from its ability to hold bones in place.

The exercises in this chapter all involve those two muscle functions: pulling bones together and holding bones stable in relation to one another. Many of the exercises involve "axial extension," or lengthening of the spine along an invisible vertical line that runs through the body's center of gravity.

Hanging in the Balance

Although the center of gravity varies in each individual, it is usually described as being midway between the heel and the bones in the top of the feet, runs just in front of the ankle bone, slightly in front of the knee joint, slightly in back of the hip joint, and directly through the center of the lumbar vertebrae. It runs through the body midway between the front and back of the chest and through the center of the vertebrae in the neck; there it passes through the earlobe and through the exact center of the head (See Illustration 7).

Imagine the body divided in half in three different ways: front to back, side to side, and top to bottom. These divisions are points of reference for anatomical movement, and are referred to as "planes." The division from front to back is called the coronal plane, because it runs along a naturally occurring fissure in the coronal bone of skull. The division of the body into right and left halves is called the sagittal plane, and the division into top half and bottom halves is referred to as the transverse plane. The intersection of all these planes is a point that runs directly through the center of the body.

Your body is subjected to the force of gravity regardless of what position it is in. When you are standing or moving, gravity pulls down on every part of you. Its invisible force puts increased pressure on the bones of your body and increased strain on the ligaments and muscles that connect your bones. When you are standing in a correctly aligned position, your muscles and bones are suspended along the invisible vertical line along which gravity pulls. Your muscles are supported by the delicate balance provided by even distribution of their weight along this invisible line and by passive tension of the ligaments in the spine. This allows you to bend, stoop, squat, recline, or lie down without undue stress or strain on the structures of your body.

Poor posture effectively means that your body weight is distributed unevenly on your skeleton. The result: increased strain on your bones, muscles, joints, ligaments, and other connective tissues. Your respiration and circulation are affected, and so is the function of the organs in your abdominal area. Overall, there is less efficient movement and less stability of your body as a whole.

Chip off the Old Block

Postural habits tend to run in families. Notice a family where the father is tall and thin, with very rounded shoulders, hips locked forward, and a sunken chest, and then look at his children. There's a good chance you'll see the same posture developing in them. Postural habits often begin during adolescence. As young girls begin to develop breasts, they often feel self-conscious and begin to slouch to hide the evidence of their development. If a girl is rapidly becoming taller than her peers, she will often compensate by hunching, particularly if she is getting taller than the boys in her class. Take a look at the teenage boys around you. Most of them are looking at their feet a good deal of the time, especially when they're around adults. I'm not sure why, but it seems to go with the territory. If an adolescent is involved in sports, theater, or dance, there is a chance they'll find role models that may change the way they stand and move, but if not, the chances are they will model their parents' postural habits.

Postural misalignment that results from abnormal skeletal development, such as scoliosis (curvature of the spine), bow-legs, or knock-knees, often do not cause pain. Because our bodies are wonderful at adapting, a person with a congenital skeletal condition often will develop a system of synergistic adaptation that prevents the other areas of the body from being overstressed in normal movement. Unfortunately, the misalignment is still there and often makes such a person more vulnerable to injury when participating in sports. When this occurs, it upsets the balance the body has developed and may initiate pain that persists and becomes chronic. The injury unmasks the deeper problems.

I worked with a young man who was the coach of a university ski team. Under his direction the team was twice named U.S. collegiate champions. He was a superb athlete, but suffered from severe pain caused by scoliosis he'd had all his life. He wrote me this letter after we had stopped our exercise sessions.

I thought my chronic back problems and pain were going to be with me the rest of my life. Because of the pain in my back, I was often unable to function as a coach and athletic trainer. The unique approach of belly breathing, deep abdominal exercises, and back exercises has completely relieved me of pain and allowed me to be aware of my inner balance. I have recently incorporated these exercises in my Alpine ski team workouts with phenomenal results.

The Same Old Song and Dance

Repetitive activity probably plays the biggest role in developing poor postural habits. Your body will adapt to any consistently repeated and prolonged position. A person who stands behind a counter for long periods may stand in a posture that rests against his or her ligaments. In other words, the knees will lock backward and the body weight will rest upon the ligaments at the back of the knee. These ligaments function as brakes to stop the knees from extending backward. In a person who stands with locked knees all day, these ligaments eventually become stretched and weakened, as do the hamstring muscles in the back of the thigh. Repeated prolonged stretching of the ligaments impairs their elasticity and then permanent lengthening occurs.

If this goes on for years, the knees may begin to rotate inward, flaring the lower leg out into a bowed position just from supporting the weight of the body. Typically, I also see these people usually thrust their hips forward so that they stand resting against the ligaments that connect the pelvis to the top of the thigh. In this case the hip flexor muscles—psoas major and minor—become overstretched and weak, and because the body is collapsing onto itself, the muscles in the chest and the front of the shoulders become adaptively shortened and pull the upper back into an overly rounded posture. As this happens, the neck must move forward, the chin lifts to bring the eyes level and . . . well, we've been down that road before.

The unfortunate conclusion of this sequential collapse of the structure is a body that looks (and feels!) like it's lacking in support, lacking in strength, and lacking in energy.

There are many other activities that create and reinforce poor posture. Someone who drives for a living, say a truck or taxi driver, or even a salesman who spends many hours on the road, will be continuously repeating and developing poor posture. They keep their lower backs in a flexed position, arms held at about chest or shoulder level, resting on the steering wheel, all of which cause the forward rolling in of the shoulders. Sitting in this flexed position allows the abdominal wall to be completely slack and to protrude. Just describing the posture makes me tired. Imagine how stressful it must be to the muscles in the neck and shoulders to sustain the arms in that position hour after hour, day after day.

Anyone sitting at a desk—working on a computer, technicians working in a hospital laboratory, architects drawing sketches on a drafting board, or students reading and writing—will duplicate the same posture. If the person is fortunate enough to have an ergonomically correct chair, he or she may experience less stress on the lower back, but the position of the arms, shoulders, and chest will be similar. In every occupation that requires looking down at a desk, the neck is subjected to severe stress.

Now, with all this talk about the negative effects of poor posture, you're probably feeling depressed, and you can see how that will affect your posture!

Illustration 130

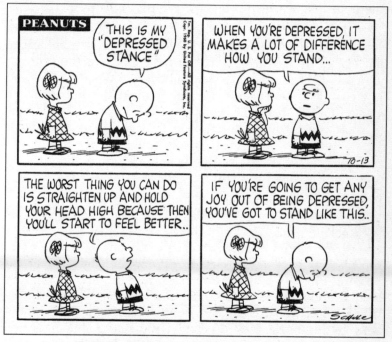

PEANUTS reprinted by permission of United Features Syndicate, Inc.

Bone(s) of Contention

Now don't get too down on yourself. There are few people who exercise all the aspects of ideal posture. Many things factor into your musculoskeletal alignment. There are variations in body type, contour, size, and proportion that affect the way the weight is distributed over your skeleton. Many variations are genetic. Genetics not only play a huge role in the way we are put together, they also affect the way we *carry* our bodies. Take a minute to observe the way your children or parents walk. Look familiar?

You'll notice a familiar pattern in gaits as well as postures. Muscle size and shape, particularly in the lower part of the body, play important roles in movement. The ability to develop muscles is strongly determined by our genetic makeup, and large muscles in the thigh and lower leg affect our gait.

So there are some things we have control over and can change and some we cannot. The goal is to reduce imbalance that causes undue stress and assist the body in returning to homeostasis or normal, healthy function. So don't run out and quit your job. Don't stop driving. Reduce the imbalance in your posture by balancing your activities. If your job or favorite sport constantly reinforces one direction of movement or static positioning, you need to integrate activity that works opposing muscle groups. Strengthening those *opposing* muscle groups is the key. I say groups because you will not achieve homeostasis by simply exercising one weak muscle. Activity must include the actions of other muscles in a way that will be therapeutic for the *whole* body.

I haven't talked much about the other changes and imbalances that occur as a result of either injury, trauma, or aging. A variety of conditions can cause either acute or chronic back pain. Bulging or herniated discs are more common than you would imagine. Research using MRIs (magnetic resonance images) on randomly selected adult subjects showed evidence that annular bulges (when the outer ring of the disc pushes out from between the vertebrae) are present in a large percentage of the population, often without accompanying pain.

If there is no direct pressure on a nerve root, there won't necessarily be pain. What causes the pain are the muscular imbalances the body experiences in trying to adapt or protect an area that has been compromised. For instance, if a disc has bulged to the right, the muscles on the left side of the spine may contract and try to pull the weight of the body away from the disc in order to prevent undue stress. This lateral shift can be very painful.

You may begin this program, even if you have sustained an injury that resulted in a herniated disc, as long as you have been released from the treatment of your primary health care provider. These exercises are also a natural follow-up to traditional physical therapy. Occasionally, traditional treatment does not bring relief. If that has happened to you, take this program very slowly, and only do those exercises that make you feel better.

Teaching an Old Dog New Tricks

The program of strengthening exercises is meant to correct faulty postural alignment by getting you to assume and sustain corrected body positions for a period of time necessary to allow the body to record and store the movement as new muscle memory. This occurs in the following way: The connection between the brain and muscle activity takes place using a system referred to as *the sensory-motor feedback loop.* The sensory nerves in the brain perceive information through our many senses, whether the information is visual, auditory, or tactile. The brain then sends information to the motor nerves for the muscles to respond with movement—your brain tells you to put your foot here instead of there, to pull your hand back from a flame, to brush your hair out of your eyes. The flow of communication is continuous.

The responses that I just listed are automatic and serve a purpose. They protect the body from stress: falling down, getting burned, or being unable to see clearly.

Most postural imbalances are caused by adaptive muscle responses to stresses that have already occurred. Such stresses could take the form of repetitive activity as discussed earlier in this chapter, or as our bodies' instincts to protect an injury. In other words, postural imbalances are learned responses. The body assumes its adapted position in order to maintain balance against the force of gravity, to bring about a level horizon to the eyes, and to ensure balance within the inner ear. These responses can be unlearned and replaced with new ones as long as those three things remain intact.

Adapting and sustaining new, corrected positions for the back, shoulders, chest, neck, and head allows the input of new sensory information into the sensory-motor feedback loop and results in new commands along the motor nerves to the muscles.

The ability of the central nervous system to absorb new information and adapt is what has allowed our species to survive and adjust to changing external conditions. By reinforcing this process as you repeat the exercises and postural repositioning consistently over several weeks, the movements become integrated at a subcortical level within your brain. You have the ability to turn a voluntary move into an involuntary move. Just as with practice you'll begin holding your abdominals in and up without thinking about it, so too you will begin to carry your back "longer." You will keep your chest lifted and open when you are standing, and you will sit up straighter. You will catch yourself when you slouch because it will no longer feel comfortable.

Although we may not be able to totally reverse all of the muscle imbalances that we've programed into our sensory-motor feedback loop, we can make significant improvements in our posture, thereby improving our functional movement. You'll actually change the way you look (and believe me, people will comment on it) and eliminate the discomfort that often accompanies poor posture. Your back will feel stronger, and it won't bother you at the end of the day. Your shoulders will appear broader, and you will look as though you have grown a couple of inches, to say nothing of the increase in your energy level.

Here's just one example of the wonders this program can work. A young woman was referred to me for exercise therapy following an acute muscle spasm that she had when lifting a heavy object into a truck. She had a severe curvature of the spine, not only in an S curve to the side, but also an extremely rounded upper back. This is what she had to report after adopting the program:

Although I inherited the curve in my back from my paternal grandmother, I have always thought of myself as stronger than the average woman. I was unaware that the strong, painfully tight muscles in my shoulders were the result of my middle back being too weak. The muscles in my whole lower left back were extremely weak, and my shoulders were curved forward. After only three of the exercise sessions, I felt my range of motion begin to increase. I felt my shoulders and chest opening up. I have learned how to stand and sit with good posture by using the muscles in my back and abdomen. Best of all is my new feeling of strength when I stand erect.

Getting Down to Brass Tacks

The following exercises should be done every other day, not every day. Because these exercises are using large muscles and more involved muscle groups than those in the previous chapters, you may experience muscle soreness a day or two after doing them. This usually happens between twenty-four and forty-eight hours after exercising, and should be gone by the third day.

Normally the affected area will feel tender when you move. Most likely you'll have this sensation in the area between your shoulder blades, but you may feel slight soreness down your whole back and in your buttocks. The most common remark I hear from people is "I can tell my back has had a workout."

Caution: If you feel any pain in your neck, shoulders, or back, discontinue the exercises. Pain is quite different from tenderness. Pain indicates that something is wrong. If pain persists beyond twenty-four hours, consult your primary health provider.

If the pain subsides after twenty-four hours, restart the program, but only do one exercise every other day. If you experience no pain by the second day, repeat the first exercise and add a second one. Follow the same procedure. Wait twenty-four hours before adding another exercise. This process of elimination will allow you to determine which exercise caused you discomfort in the first place. Remember, not every exercise is right for every person. You may have a specific condition that would be exacerbated by one particular exercise but that doesn't mean you can't do the others.

A physical therapist whose course I once took said that exercise is as stressful to the body as injury. That stress is what causes a chemical response in the body to make a muscle larger and stronger. The key is controlling the amount of stress.

He was right. Exercise is meant to be stressful to the specific muscles you are targeting for strengthening. Making muscles work harder than they normally do is what elicits that strengthening response. But it is controlled stress—small amounts of stress, for a small amount of time. Too much stress results in injury and a tearing down of the muscles rather than a building up.

So, go slowly. Listen to your body. When you have worked your way through all the exercises, begin to do the ones that work for you three times a week. Just as with the abdominal strengthening program, consistency is important if you want to reeducate your muscles. If you are faithful about doing them for a few months, you will see that your body has adapted new ways of holding itself. You will walk, stand, and sit differently. When that happens you can drop down to a maintenance program of once or twice a week. Just remember, if your daily activity mainly consists of sustaining forward motion for long periods, you will need to balance that with activity for the opposing muscle groups, so you may need to continue to do a few of these exercises every other day to maintain postural balance. For this purpose, at the end of this chapter there is a list of exercise combinations that you can easily integrate into your daily schedule.

Many of these exercises are stretches as well as strengtheners. When you inhale, the muscles in the front of the body expand and stretch. On the exhale, muscles in the back relax and may lengthen. We are going to use that principle to open the chest area while we are strengthening the muscles in the back. This is a very effective method of improving your posture by reprogramming your muscles while you breathe deeply. It's also a great way to release stress from the body and quiet the mind.

All of the exercises have the *slow release* component. Muscle tissue is highly elastic and any movement done quickly, either lengthening or shortening, will have a recoil response if you release too quickly. By releasing out of either a contraction or a stretch slowly (I call it "sneaking out"), you reduce the recoil response and allow the muscles to retain the new muscle memory of the corrected position. With each repetition, the recoil response diminishes until your body maintains the corrected position even at rest.

Note: Inhale on each lift or movement, exhale on any curl forward, and breathe normally during the holding stage. Always return to deep belly breathing between repetitions. *If you are pregnant, and past your first trimester, do not do the prone (stomach-lying) exercises.* As long as they do not cause you discomfort, all the other exercises are great for you.

Exercise 40 Bench-Seated Wall Press with Breath

Position a bench or stool about an inch from the wall. Sit on it with your buttocks pressed up closely against the wall and your feet flat on the floor. The top of your legs should be level with or just below your hips (adjust the height of your bench accordingly). Place your arms against the wall at a slight diagonal down from the shoulder, palms facing out (Illustration 131). **Put your shoulder blades firmly against the wall and press down and back with the tops of your shoulders, and don't let any part of your shoulders lose contact with the wall.** *Do not try to hold your head against the wall;* instead think about moving the back of your neck toward the wall. Your head should stay in line with your neck. This may be an uncomfortable position at first. Close your eyes and breathe in slowly through your nose, feeling the front of your chest stretch open as you inhale. **Keep pressing your shoulders down and back.** Relax the muscles in your back and neck as you breathe out through your mouth (Illustration 132). Repeat this several times, trying to let your body relax in this position. Relax completely and assume your normal sitting posture.

Illustration 131

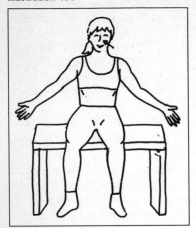

Illustration 132

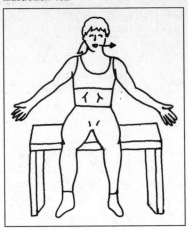

Bench-Seated Wall Press with Breath

❖ *Special Tips*
If you do not have a bench, use a flat-bottomed, straight-backed chair.

Exercise 41 Bench-Seated Arm Raise with Breath

Position a bench or stool about an inch from the wall. Sit on it with your buttocks pressed up closely against the wall and your feet flat on the floor. The tops of your legs should be level with or just below your hips (adjust the height of your bench accordingly). Place your arms against the wall at a slight diagonal down from the shoulders, palms facing out (Illustration 133). Put your shoulder blades firmly against the wall and press down and back with the tops of your shoulders, but don't let any part of your shoulders lose contact with the wall. *Do not try to hold your head against the wall;* instead think about moving the back of your neck toward the wall. Your head should stay in line with your neck. Close your eyes and breathe in slowly through your nose, feeling the front of your chest stretch open as you inhale. **As you inhale, slowly slide your extended arms up to shoulder height (do this** in small steps), **keeping your back and arms in contact with the wall.** *Only move your arms as you inhale.* When you complete each inhalation, stop moving your arms and exhale, relaxing your back in that position (Illustration 134). Keep gently pressing your shoulders down and back. **When you inhale again, continue moving your arms until they are level with the tops of your shoulders** (Illustration 135). Take as many breaths as you need to reach this position. **Move slowly.** When you have reached the top, hold for a count of four as you breathe. Release and return to your normal sitting posture. Relax completely.

Repeat 1 time only.

Illustration 133   Illustration 134   Illustration 135

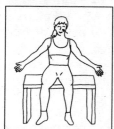 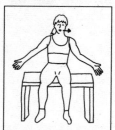 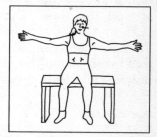

Bench-Seated Arm Raise with Breath

The next two exercises are also stretch and strengthening moves that are both challenging and a little uncomfortable at first. Do your best to achieve the positions I've described. Your body will loosen up, and the exercises will become easier with each repetition. The important thing to remember is *not to alter or change your body position* after you have released the tension. When you relax slowly, your body will make its own adjustments. If you actively alter your position to one that *feels* comfortable you will lose the cumulative benefits of these stretches. These are intentionally exaggerated positions. The purpose is to reeducate the muscles in the back and chest so that your body will adapt a modified version when you are standing or sitting.

Note: If your neck is more comfortable being supported,

use a small rolled towel or pillow. If you have been diagnosed as having a military neck—one that has lost its curve—do not stretch your neck into the floor. Instead, allow it to remain relaxed throughout the back-lying exercises

Exercise 42 Supine Shoulder Blade Squeeze

On the floor, lie on your back with a pillow under your knees and your arms at your sides. Pull your chin in and down and lengthen the back of your neck toward the floor (Illustration 136). Pull your abdominals **in and up** and contract your buttocks. **Slowly rotate your lower back toward the floor** (Illustration 137). **Roll your shoulders back, rotating your arms around until the backs of your hands are on the floor** (Illustration 138). Keep your abdominals held in tightly and increase the pelvic tilt. Inhale deeply through your nose, and as you exhale through your mouth, **pull your shoulder blades together and press them down.** Hold in that position focusing on your breathing. **In-**

Illustration 136

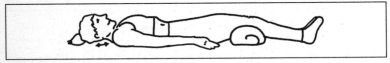

Illustration 137

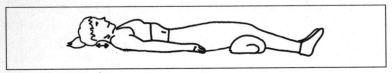

Illustration 138

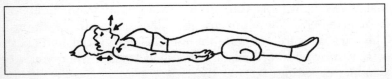

Supine Shoulder Blade Squeeze

crease your pelvic tilt, keeping your back flat against the floor. **Stretch the back of your neck toward the floor.** Hold for a slow count of four, breathing easily through your nose, and **slowly release.** Don't alter your position; simply allow the tension to leave your body. Begin your next repetition from that starting position.

Repeat 4 times.

Exercise 43 Shoulder Blade Squeeze with External Arm Rotation

On the floor, lie on your back with a pillow under your knees and your arms extended to either side, palms down. Pull your chin in and down and lengthen the back of your neck toward the floor. Pull your abdominals **in and up** and **contract** your buttocks. **Slowly rotate your lower back toward the floor.** Roll your shoulders back until the backs of your hands are on the floor (Illustration 139). Make relaxed fists with your hands and bend your elbows to 90-degree angles, with the knuckles facing the ceiling (Illustration 140). Inhale deeply through your nose, and as you exhale through your mouth, **pull your shoulder blades together and press them down, rotating your arms out and moving your thumbs toward the floor** (Illustration 141). Move slowly, focus on your breathing, and go as far as your range of motion will allow you to go. Increase your pelvic tilt and keep your back flat against the floor. Stretch the back of your neck toward the floor. Hold for a slow count of four, breathing easily through

Illustration 139

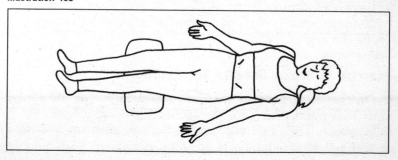

Illustration 140

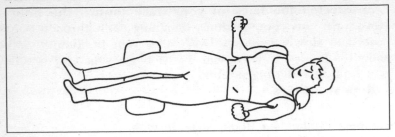

Illustration 141

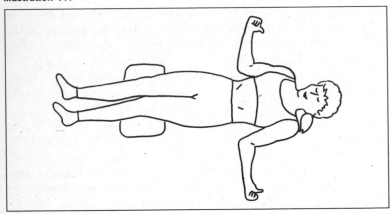

Shoulder Blade Squeeze with External Arm Rotation

your nose, and **slowly release.** Don't alter your position; simply allow the tension to leave your body. Return your arms to their starting position and begin your next repetition.

Repeat 4 times.

If this exercise bothers your shoulders, skip this one and go on to the next.

Exercise 44 Supine Butterfly Arm Pull-Down

On the floor, lie on your back with a pillow or roll under your knees and your arms in the butterfly position, palms up (Illustration 142). Pull your abdominals **in and up** and do a strong pelvic tilt. Inhale deeply through your nose, and as you exhale through your mouth, **press your shoulders down toward your hips, sliding your shoulder blades down with the muscles in the back** (Illustration 143). *Keep your arms on the floor.* Do not allow your back to arch up off the floor. Hold for a slow count of four, breathing easily through your nose. Then **slowly release.** Don't alter your position; simply allow the tension to leave your body. Begin your next repetition from that starting position.

Repeat 4 times.

Illustration 142

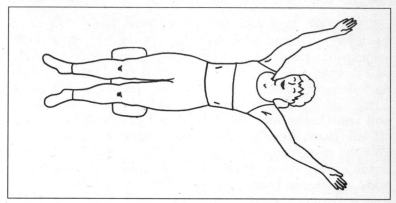

Illustration 143

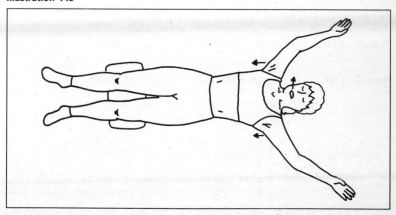

Supine Butterfly Arm Pull-Down

❖ *Special Tips*

Keep your arms extended, and try not to let the elbows bend. Don't slide your arms down; just think of pulling the bottom of your shoulder blades down toward your hips.

I know you've done this next stretch before, but it's a perfect way to release the tension in your back after the last two exercises.

Exercise 45 Double Bent-Knee Body Curl

Lie on your back with your knees bent. Lift your feet off the floor and bring your knees up into a 90-degree angle, holding the outside of your knees with your hands. Allow the legs to open wide to stretch the buttocks (Illustration 144). Find a neutral place with your lower back and rest there. Inhale deeply through your nose, and as you exhale, **slowly pull your knees into your chest and gently lift your hips off the floor, keeping the knees apart** (Illustration 145). Feel the stretch in your lower back area. Inhale deeply, and as you exhale, **slowly tuck your chin and curl your upper body up toward your knees** (Illustration 146). Feel the stretch in your upper and midback. Gently lower your upper body, keeping your knees pulled to your chest. *Stop and allow the back to relax.* Slowly lower the hips to the floor, but keep hold of your knees. Find a neutral place with your back. Slowly lower your feet to the floor and allow your back to

Illustration 144

Illustration 145

Illustration 146

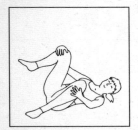
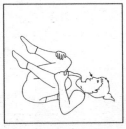
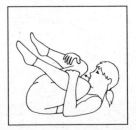

Double Bent-Knee Body Curl

relax. Extend your legs over your rolled towel or pillow. Completely relax and belly-breathe.

Repeat 1 time.

This stretch is repeated several times throughout the program. If it does not feel comfortable, or is difficult to do, you may substitute the Single Knee to Chest Stretch described in the next chapter.

❖ *Special Tips*

If curling up your upper body is too difficult, proceed with the rest of the instructions without lifting your upper body.

The next four exercises actively strengthen all three areas of the trapezius muscle in the back. By changing the position of the arms for each lift, we isolate specific parts of the muscle as we alter the resistance. The part of the muscle being "loaded" is determined by where the arms are in relation to your torso.

Exercise 46 Prone Back Lift 1

Lie on your stomach with your forehead on the floor or supported on a small rolled towel. Move your arms so they're fully extended over your head (Illustration 147). Pull your abdominals **in and up, contract your buttocks,** and **do a pelvic tilt.** Keep your forehead on the floor and slowly raise your

Illustration 147

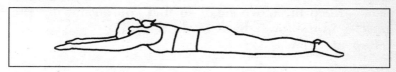

Illustration 148

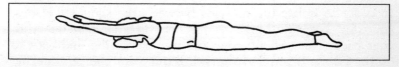

Prone Back Lift 1

arms about 2 inches off the floor (Illustration 148). *Keep the lift small.* Hold for a slow count of four, breathing easily through your nose, and keep the muscles in your neck relaxed. **Slowly lower your arms** and relax completely.
    Repeat 4 times.

❖ *Special Tips*
    If this exercise causes you any strain in your neck, don't do it. Although this is a great strengthener, if you have had a whiplash injury or history of cervical problems, this may not be an appropriate exercise for you.

Exercise 47 Prone Back Lift 2

Lie on your stomach with your forehead on the floor or supported on a small rolled towel. Place your arms 90 degrees from your shoulders, with your palms down (Illustration 149). Your head, neck, and spine should all be aligned. Keep your chin slightly tucked. Pull your abdominals **in and up, contract your buttocks,** and do a pelvic tilt. Keep the tops of your feet on the floor. Inhale deeply through your nose, and as you exhale, lift your chest, head, and arms as a unit, *raising them no more than 2 inches* off the floor (Illustration 150). The backs of your hands and elbows should lift and remain level with each other. *The back of your head should remain level with your back.* Hold your body in a lifted position for a slow count of four, breathing easily through your nose. **Slowly lower** your upper body to the floor and relax completely. **Keep the move small so that you do not use the muscles in the lower back to do the lift.**
    Repeat 4 times.

❖ *Special Tips*
    Make sure you do not lift your chin as you do this exercise. In order to isolate the muscles between the shoulder blades, you must keep the back of your neck in a straight line with your back. Think about using the muscles in the mid-back to do the lifting. If you find yourself lifting your chin, try tucking it slightly.

Illustration 149

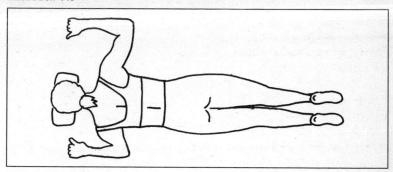

Illustration 150

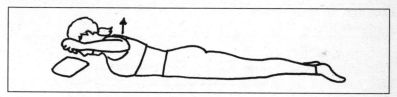

Prone Back Lift 2

Exercise 48 Prone Butterfly Arm Lift

Lie on your stomach with your forehead on the floor or supported on a small rolled towel. Extend your arms diagonally about 45 degrees from your shoulders, palms facing down (Illustration 151). Your head, neck, and spine should be in alignment. Keep your chin slightly tucked. Pull your abdominals **in and up, contract your buttocks,** and **do a pelvic tilt** to stabilize the lumbar spine. Inhale deeply through your nose, and as you exhale through your mouth, **lift your arms from the floor about 2 inches and slide your shoulder blades down your back** (Illustrations 152 and 153). *Do not lift your head.* Hold for a slow count of four, breathing easily through your nose. **Slowly** lower to the floor and release. Return to your starting position and relax completely.

Repeat 4 times.

Illustration 151

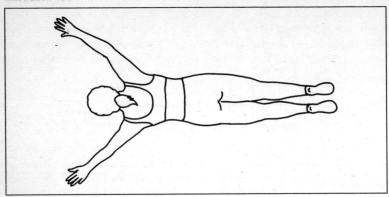

Illustration 152

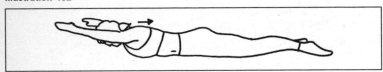

Illustration 153

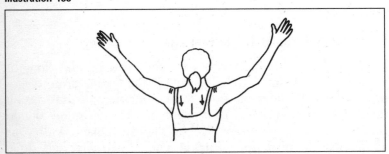

Prone Butterfly Arm Lift

❖ *Special Tips*

This exercise isolates the lower portion of the trapezius. One of the functions of this muscle is to hold the bottom of the scapula firmly against the back when the arms are lifted. This area is a weak spot for many people and contributes to "winged" scapula. The key is to keep your elbows extended while moving your arms. The emphasis is on pulling the shoulder blades down your back, not together. Your arms will automatically move as you slide your shoulder blades down, and you should feel this at the bottom of your scapula. Keep your arms straight, and at the end of each lift, reposition them.

Exercise 49 Prone Shoulder Blade Squeeze

Lie on your stomach with your forehead on the floor or supported on a small rolled towel. Your arms should be at your sides with the backs of your hands on the floor (Illustration 154). Your head, neck, and spine should all be in alignment. Keep your chin slightly tucked. Pull **in and up** with your abdominals, **contract your buttocks,** and **do a pelvic tilt.** Keep the tops of your feet on the floor. Inhale deeply through your nose, and as you exhale through your mouth, **pull your shoulder blades together and slide them down** (Illustration 155). Hold for a slow count of four, breathing easily through your nose. *Do not lift your head.* Keep the

Illustration 154

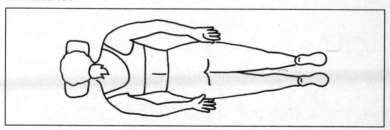

Illustration 155

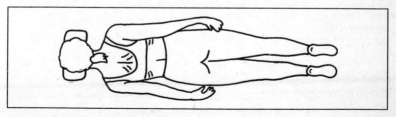

Prone Shoulder Blade Squeeze

muscles in the back of your neck relaxed. **Release slowly** and allow your shoulders to return to the starting position. Relax completely. Keep your pelvis tilted throughout the move.

Repeat 4 times.

Exercise 50 Prone Back Lift 3

Lie on your stomach with your forehead on the floor or supported on a small rolled towel. Your arms at your sides with the back of your hands on the floor (Illustration 156). Your head, neck, and spine should all be in alignment. Keep your chin slightly tucked. Pull **in and up** with your abdominals, **contract your buttocks,** and **do a pelvic tilt.** Keep the top of your feet on the floor. Inhale deeply through your nose, and as you exhale through your mouth, lift your head, neck, and chest as a unit; *raising no higher than 2 inches* off the floor (Illustration 157). Hold for a slow count of four, breathing easily through your nose. **Slowly lower** and relax completely. **Keep the move small so that you do not use the muscles in your lower back to do the lift.**

Repeat 4 to 6 times.

Illustration 156

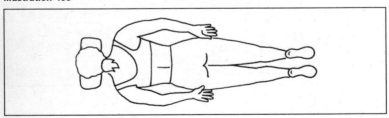

Illustration 157

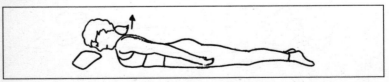

Prone Back Lift 3

Exercise 51 Cat Back Stretch Combo

Position yourself on your hands and knees. Your arms should be directly under your shoulders and your knees a comfortable distance apart. Inhale deeply through your nose, and as you exhale, **tuck your chin, push up off your hands,** and **fully round your back** (Illustration 158). Hold long enough to feel the muscles stretch, breathing easily through your nose. Gently push your ribs out to the right and to the left, holding until you feel the stretch (Illustrations 159 and 160). Inhale deeply again, and as you exhale **slowly lower your back, raise your chin,** and **tilt your buttocks up,** allowing the midback to gently drop into a "sagging bridge." Feel the shoulder blades move together (Illustration 161). Slowly lower your hips back onto your heels. *Allow the knees to spread wide apart.* Place your forehead on the floor and stretch your arms out in front of you as far as you can with your palms down (Illustration 162). Hold until you feel the stretch down the sides of the back, breathing easily through your nose. Then move back up onto your hands and knees and repeat the sequence one more time.

If you are not able to sit back on your heels, or that

Illustration 158

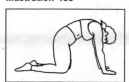

Illustration 159

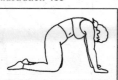

Illustration 160

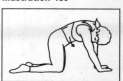

Illustration 161

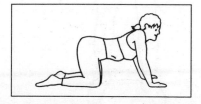

Illustration 162

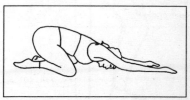

Cat Back Stretch Combo

portion of the stretch stresses your back, only do the cat back and sagging bridge.

The following exercise is great for strengthening the muscles of the upper back (the middle and lower trapezius muscles), and correcting an overaccentuated curve in the lower back. It is most effective because you are applying the principle of pulling in and up with your abdominal muscles while in a weight-bearing position, as you will now do in your normal everyday activity. This exercise will create new postural muscle memory most effectively if you do it at least once each day.

Exercise 52 Wall Standing

Stand with your heels 8 to 10 inches from a wall. Place your hips, middle back, and shoulder blades against the wall (Illustration 163). *Try to pull the back of your neck toward*

Illustration 163   **Illustration 164**

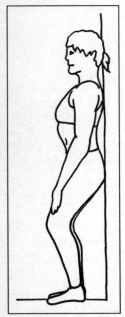
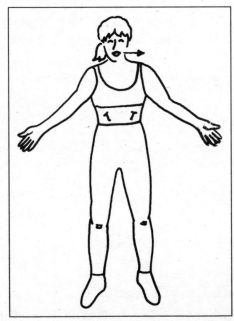

Illustration 165   **Illustration 166**

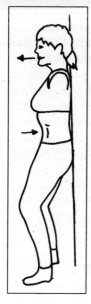
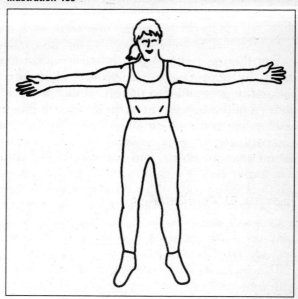

Wall Standing

the wall, not your head. Bend your knees slightly and place
your hands against the wall diagonally downward from the
shoulder, with the palms facing forward (Illustration 164). Inhale deeply through your nose, allowing your midsection to
expand. Exhale through your mouth and pull your abdominals
in and up (Illustration 165). Focus on pulling in strongly with
the muscles in the lower abdomen and allow your pelvis to
rotate forward, moving your lower back toward the wall. Go
back to breathing easily through your nose. Hold your abdominals **in and up tightly, and slowly slide your arms up to
shoulder height,** keeping the backs of your arms and hands
against the wall (Illustration 166). If the arm slide causes discomfort in your shoulder area, keep your arms at hip level for
a slow count of four. Lower your arms to the starting position.
Slowly release your abdominals and relax.

   Do 1 or 2 repetitions.

✤ *Special Tips*
Some of my clients experience discomfort as they practice this one. Concentrate on relaxing your neck and breathing.

You have just completed the structured strengthening program. In order to achieve maximum benefits, you should do the entire program two or three times a week. Each position is as important as the next, so don't skip any exercises unless they cause you pain or discomfort. By the end of a month you will see an improvement in your posture (people may even comment on it), and you should *feel* different. You will feel looser and able to move with greater ease. You may actually feel taller and lighter on your feet. As you continue with the program and begin to integrate the improved posture into your functional movement, you may modify the program and only do those exercises that you enjoy the most or that you feel are most beneficial.

I've included the following exercises for variety. They use different starting positions to work the muscles in the back. You may use them in place of any exercise in the structured program, add them to your routine, or do them on alternate days.

The next two exercises isolate those deep muscles in the back that attach vertebrae to vertebrae. Remember how the spine is able to move in segments? Well, these exercises force your spine to do just that do just that. By coming up *one vertebra at a time* each muscle is worked individually. These exercises are wonderful at stretching the spine and strengthening it. Exercises 54 through 58 are excellent for strengthening the upper body if you are pregnant. The Wall Push-up is particularly good for keeping the muscles in the chest toned.

Exercise 53 Seated C Curl-up

Sit on the floor with your knees bent and your feet flat on the floor. Sit up tall on your buttocks and clasp your hands around the outside of your knees. Lower your chin all the way down onto your chest and allow your back to round into a C position (Illustration 167). Your arms should be fully extended with your body weight supported by your hands gripping your knees. Completely relax into this position. Moving **very slowly, begin to straighten the spine into an upright position by pulling your abdominals in and up and using the muscles in your back.** Come up one vertebrae at a time, breathing easily through your nose (Illustration 168). *Do not pull yourself up with your arms.* Keep your chin lowered, and as you straighten up, open the chest area by keeping your shoulders dropped down and rolled back. When your back is fully erect, raise your chin, lengthen the back of your neck, and stretch up as tall as you can (Illustration 169). Hold for a count of four. **Slowly release** and completely relax.

Repeat 2 times.

Illustration 167

Illustration 168

Illustration 169

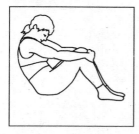
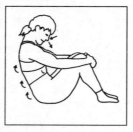
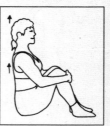

Seated C Curl-up

✤ *Special Tips*

Make sure you keep your chin down on your chest and your shoulders dropped throughout the exercise. Lifting your head and stretching up tall is the last thing you do to complete the stretch.

Exercise 54 Standing Roll-up Shoulder Shrug

Stand with your feet hip width apart and your knees slightly bent. Let your chin drop onto your chest and bend forward from the waist with your arms hanging down directly in front of you. Let your upper and middle back curl into a C. *Do not*

curl the lower back. The bend is from the waist, not the hips.
Exhale slowly through your mouth as you tuck your pelvis
forward and let your whole upper body relax and hang (Illustration 170). Your lower back should still be straight, not bent.
On your inhalation, **slowly** count to four as you roll up, one
vertebra at a time, until your back is erect. On the count of
four, lift your head and shrug your shoulders (Illustration 171),
rolling them *back and down* (Illustration 172). Then bend
forward and roll back down to a count of four.

Repeat 4 times.

Illustration 170   Illustration 171   Illustration 172

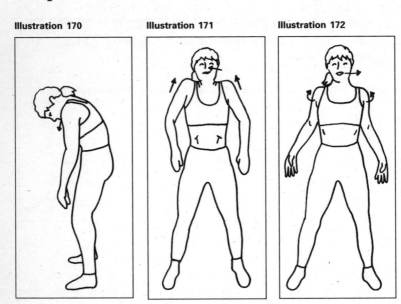

Standing Roll-up Shoulder Shrug

✤ *Special Tips*

Make sure you keep your chin down on your chest until
your back is fully erect. Lift your head just as you begin your
shrug. Look at the illustration carefully. Make sure you don't
round your lower back.

Exercise 55 Overhead Wall Press

Stand facing a wall, with your feet 15 to 18 inches away from it. Your feet are together, heels flat on the floor. Place your hands on the wall as high as you can, thumbs touching, fingers pointing straight up (Illustration 173). Pull your abdominals **in and up and contract your buttocks.** *Relax the tops of your shoulders. Let them drop.* **Slowly lower your body toward the wall until your forearms, nose, forehead, and chest touch it** (Illustration 174). Keep your heels flat on the floor. (If you can't, just move your feet closer to the wall). Individual range of motion within the shoulder joint

Illustration 173

Illustration 174

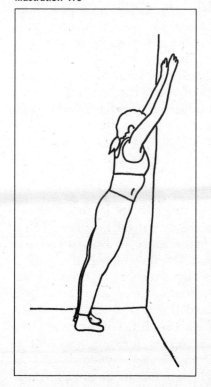
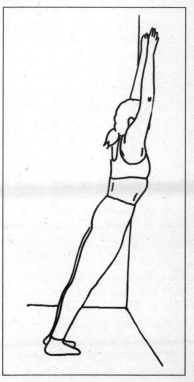

Overhead Wall Press

will determine how far you are able to go. Push your body back to the original position by pressing against the wall with your palms. Inhale deeply through your nose on the lowering move and exhale slowly through your mouth as you push off. **Repeat 4 to 6 times.**

❖ *Special Tips*
The purpose of this exercise is to isolate the lower trapezius muscle in the back. This muscle is weakened on many people. One of its primary functions is to stabilize your shoulder blades when you raise your arms. Though you will feel all the muscles in your back working, you should be especially aware of tension in the muscles at the bottom of your shoulder blades. *Do not let your body sag in the middle.* Keeping your abdominals in and up will allow you to lower your body as a unit. Bend forward from your ankles not your waist.

The next two exercises work the muscles in your arms and chest as well as the muscles in your back. The starting position isolates the muscles that pull the shoulder blades together and stabilizes them during movement.

Exercise 56 Wide-Arm Wall Press

Stand facing a wall, with your feet 15 to 18 inches away from it. Your feet are together, heels flat on the floor. Place your hands on the wall as high as you can, but spread the arms so that your thumbs are just above eye level (Illustration 175), fingers pointing at the ceiling. Pull your abdominals **in and up** and **contract your buttocks.** *Relax your shoulders.* **Slowly lower your body toward the wall until your fore-arms, nose, forehead, and chest touch it** (Illustration 176). Push back to your original position by pressing against the wall with your palms. Inhale deeply through your nose as you lower and exhale slowly through your mouth as you push off. **Repeat 4 to 6 times.**

Illustration 175

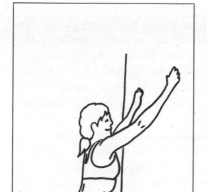

Illustration 176

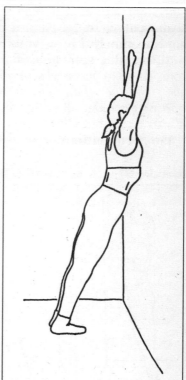

Wide-Arm Wall Press

✤ *Special Tips*

If you have restricted motion in your shoulder area, this may not be a comfortable exercise for you. Try it, lowering halfway to the wall, then push back. If this action still causes you discomfort, do not do this exercise.

Exercise 57 Wall Push-up

Stand facing a wall with your feet close together and about 15 inches away from the wall. Place your hands on the wall at chest level, with your fingers pointing in, your elbows out

(Illustration 177). Adjust your distance from the wall for your body and arm length. Pull your abdominals in and up and keep your chest raised and chin level. **Bending from the ankles, slowly lower your body, as a unit, toward the wall, keeping your heels flat on the floor.** Attempt to touch your chest to the backs of your hands (Illustration 178). *Do not go farther than your strength allows.* Push back to your starting position, allowing the muscles between the shoulder blades to stretch (Illustration 179).

Do 8 repetitions, 2 or 3 times.

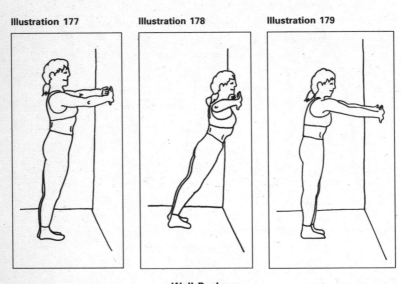

Illustration 177   Illustration 178   Illustration 179

Wall Push-up

❖ *Special Tips*
This is a real strength move for your chest, shoulders, and the backs of your upper arms. *Keep your shoulders relaxed* as you do this exercise. The tendency is to hold them up and create unnecessary tension in the neck.

Exercise 58 Standing 90-Degree External Arm Rotation

Stand with your feet about shoulder width apart, arms at your sides. Lift your ribs up out of your hips and consciously lengthen your spine. **Pull your abdominals in and up and contract your buttocks.** Bend your elbows up at a 90-degree angle from the waist, with the insides of your elbows close to your body. Curl your hands into loose fists, with your thumbs up and palms facing each other (Illustration 180). As you inhale deeply through your nose, **slowly** rotate your shoulders back, moving your arms out to your sides, keeping the 90-degree angle, with your thumbs up. Your palms will be facing forward at the end of your opening move (Illustration 181). Feel your chest open up as you inhale, and **press down and back with your shoulders** (Illustration 182). Exhale through your mouth and **slowly move your arms back into their starting position.**

Repeat 8 times. Do 3 sets, resting in between.

Illustration 180   **Illustration 181**   **Illustration 182**

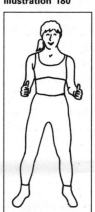
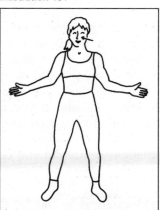
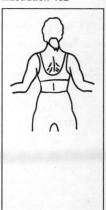

Standing 90-Degree External Arm Rotation

Exercise Combinations for the Work day

10:00 A.M. break: Exercise 34 Bench Squats, *followed by*
                              Exercise 35 Seated Gluteal Squeezes
12:00 P.M./lunch break: Exercise 40 Bench-Seated Wall Press with Breath, *or*

	Exercise 52 Wall Standing, *followed by*
	Exercise 55 Overhead Wall Press
3:00 P.M. break:	Exercise 57 Wall Push-up (1 set)
	Exercise 54 Standing Roll-up Shoulder Shrug, *followed by*
	Exercise 58 Standing 90-Degree Arm External Rotation (1 set)
End of workday:	Exercise 31 Standing Single-Leg Knee Bend, *followed by*
	Exercise 77 Standing Hamstring Stretch (chapter 9)
	Exercise 82 Standing Chest and Shoulder Stretch (chapter 9)
	Exercise 83 Standing or Seated Neck Stretch (chapter 9)

These combinations, or any parts of them, are great whether you have a desk job or one that involves a lot of driving. Either on your scheduled breaks or at intervals when you are able, find a wall, a chair, or a step and do the exercises that require those items. If your work environment doesn't have any of those things readily available, or you feel too conspicuous, simply do the exercises that require no equipment, such as 54, 58, 83, and 84. If you are unable to do Exercises 31 and 78 at work, I strongly recommend you do them when you get home.

A young woman was referred to me by the chiropractor I work closely with. She had been in a serious automobile accident and had struggled with debilitating headaches for weeks. She had always worked out and considered herself strong and fit. After the accident, her range of motion in both her neck and shoulders was severely limited. She was weak and rundown. She wrote me this letter after only a few weeks on my program:

I was involved in a head-on collision earlier this year. After months of severe headaches, back and neck pain, stiff-

ness, and fatigue, I began chiropractic treatment and exercise therapy. Your range of motion, back, and abdominal exercises have made my back and neck strong and pain free. The headaches are gone and my balance and stamina have improved, thus my daily workouts have never been better. I will continue these exercises throughout my life as part of my regular exercise program.

The next chapter is one of my favorites. It leads you through a series of stretches, a few of which you have been introduced to already. Some are dynamic or moving stretches and some are static or held-position stretches. There are many ways to stretch, and each lengthens the muscle fibers a little differently. So get ready to reward yourself for your hard work with some relaxing and rejuvenating stretches.

PART IV

Stretching Program

8

Moving into the
Home Stretch

Why is it that whenever we have been sitting too long in one position, or wake up in the morning or from a nap, we feel the need to stretch? Have you noticed your cat always does the same thing? It is the nature of the muscles to crave movement. Muscle are contractile tissues. In other words, the primary function of muscle tissue is to produce movement.

Muscle tissue is composed of individual muscle fibers that are made up of smaller units called *myofibrils*. These myofibrils enable the muscle to contract or shorten, and lengthen or stretch. These processes are achieved by chemical changes within the *myofilaments*, individual filaments inside the myofibrils. It's not terribly important for you to understand the micromuscle mechanics, just that muscles contract by a *sliding* action of one myofilament over another—like the action of a telescope or a radio antenna.

When a muscle is fully contracted, its length decreases from 20 to 50 percent. When passively stretched, it may lengthen to about 120 percent of its normal resting length. Muscle fibers cannot lengthen or stretch by themselves. There must be a force exerted from outside the muscle, either the force of gravity, the force of motion, the force of an opposing muscle, or the force provided by something other than your own body, such as another person or special equipment.

Muscles cannot contract of their own accord either. They

are completely dependent on impulses from the central nervous system. Without a nerve impulse, a muscle cannot contract or shorten. Paralysis occurs when the communication between the nerve and the muscle has been interrupted, either by trauma, as in a spinal cord or brain injury, or by disease.

Stretching—The Truth

So how does stretching occur? Well, there are stretch receptors called muscle spindles located in every muscle in your body. They are slender fibers encased in a tube of connective tissue and they run parallel to muscle fibers that contract. When a muscle detects a stretching force, its receptors experience a stimulus or a change in their environment. In response, they send a message through the central nervous system to the spinal nerves, which in turn send a signal to the muscle to allow the muscle fibers to lengthen.

During a stretch, the muscle goes through a series of relaxation and contraction stages, depending on what message the spindles are sending to the nerves. The duration and intensity of the stimulus determines what stage the muscle is in. For instance, when a muscle is first stretched it will allow some lengthening of the muscle fibers, but as the intensity and duration of the stretch increases, the muscle spindles experience excessive tension, and the muscle fibers contract, shortening the muscle, to take the stress off of the spindles. This is known as the stretch reflex. It is a defense mechanism of the central nervous system to avoid overstretching and to prevent muscle-tendon injuries. If the stretch is slow and gentle, the stretch reflex, in turn, will be slow and gentle.

Muscles operate in pairs, so that when one is contracting, the muscle that works in opposition to it automatically relaxes. This is known as *reciprocal innervation*. This tandem action allows movement. If the opposing muscle pulled against the contraction of the first, no movement would occur. For example, when you bend your knee back, your hamstrings (muscles in the back of the thigh) pull the leg up in back; the quadriceps (muscles in the front of the thigh) must relax for this to happen. The quadriceps normally straighten the leg. If both muscles contracted at once, the leg wouldn't move at all.

A second muscle receptor, called the Golgi Tendon Organ (GTO), serves a different function. GTOs are located at the end of each muscle, where the muscle becomes tendon and attaches to the bone. GTOs are sensitive to both muscle contraction and muscle stretch, although they cannot distinguish between the two. When they feel too much tension in the tendinous attachment, they send a signal to the muscle to relax. That's why you need to hold a static stretch for at least 30 seconds. Although the timing varies among individuals, it takes that long for the GTO to send its message to relax, and then you can usually stretch the muscle a little farther.

In turn, this additional stretching causes an automatic contraction of the opposing or antagonist muscle and prevents either muscle from being overstretched.

The Pause That Refreshes

The purpose of this stretching section is not only to increase and maintain range of motion within the joint and to bring the muscles into a more balanced relationship to one another, but also to promote relaxation. Relaxation is different from stretching. It occurs when there is no nerve impulse signal being sent to the muscle. Muscular relaxation is the cessation of tension within the muscle. Muscles that are habitually tense have a reduced supply of blood, oxygen, and other essential nutrients in their tissues. These tense muscles accumulate toxins and waste products that result in muscle soreness and chronic tenderness.

Relaxation comes *after* the muscle has been either contracted or stretched. In a relaxed state the muscles, in fact the whole body, truly rests.

The following stretches are slow, rhythmic, and continuous *moving* stretches designed to gently increase your range of motion and elongate the tissues in multidirectional positions. They allow your body to establish its own pace and degree of elasticity. Because they are *moving* rather than static stretches, they create *functional* flexibility.

The moving stretch allows the muscle spindle cells, located in the belly of the muscle, to monitor the changes in the muscle length and the speed with which those changes occur. If the muscle were lengthened too quickly, the spindle cell would respond by initiating the stretch reflex. The reflex would signal the muscle to contract, thereby resisting any further stretching. The slow, continuous movement involved in the moving stretches lengthens the muscle so gradually that the stretch reflex is postponed. You'll be able to stretch targeted muscle groups gently and safely.

The principles of slow conscious breathing, slow movement throughout the stretch, and gradual release of tension in the body described in the previous chapters apply here, too.

Visualizing your body "letting go," and allowing the body to move in the direction of the stretch, rather than pulling it into the position, stretches the body naturally and gently. With slow, continuous, and sustained movement, your joints will be stretched through their entire range of motion and become lubricated in the process.

Our muscles are layered on top of each other at oblique angles and are separated by layers of connective tissue called fascia. Alternating the direction of the arms, legs, neck, and pelvis, and moving these body parts in opposition to one another, stretches the body diagonally as well as horizontally and vertically. This creates functional pliability and flexibility in your muscle tissues.

It's important to recognize that our body's capabilities vary from day to day. Some days you feel loose and supple, other days you feel stiff and sore. The following stretching programs allow your body to tell you what it is able to do each day. By tuning in to the messages your body gives you as you begin and move through the stretches, you greatly reduce the risk of overstretching or tearing a muscle, and you'll avoid straining the connective tissue.

Your breathing, as always, plays an important role. Respiration is a complex process. When you inhale, many muscles that assist in inspiration expand. As you exhale, they relax, and other muscles, like the transversus abdominis, contract. This process will assist you as you do the moving stretches. Because the stretches may take varying amounts of time for different individuals, remember to breathe throughout the stretch and allow your body to set its own rhythm. You will practice a moderate form of the Active Belly Breathing (see page 46) as you perform these. As you release into each stretch, exhale slowly. Inhale deeply as you use your muscles to move your body back to neutral. On any stretch that involves a curl and an extension, time your breathing so that you *exhale* on the curl, gently pulling your abdominal wall *in*. *Inhale* as you extend, and let your belly relax and stretch. If you're required to hold a position for a moment, breathe naturally but deeply and slowly.

The gentle pumping motion of active breathing encourages movement in the entire spine, stimulates the flow of both cranial and spinal fluids, and massages the organs and abdominal viscera. The result is improved respiratory, organ, and brain function. The ultimate benefit is improved overall health and well-being.

Easy as Rolling off a Log

The stretches are listed in a logical progression—you start on your back, then roll to one side, onto your stomach, over to the other side, and finally end on your back again. This progression was designed to make the series, as a whole, easy to follow. If you can remember the progression of the starting positions, you'll be cued to move from one exercise into the next and won't spend unnecessary time moving around and adjusting your body.

Because you may not be able to do all the stretches every day, and because some stretches will simply not feel good to some people, you need not do them all. Identify which stretches *feel* good to you and do them in the order that *feels* best to you.

You can't really do these stretches too slowly as long as you keep moving and don't stay too long in any one position, but you can do them too quickly. Don't rush through them. That will defeat their purpose. Set aside 20 minutes every day to spend time with someone you care about—*you!*

In addition to functionally stretching the muscles and connective tissues, and lubricating and increasing range of motion in the joints, these exercises are a pleasurable and effective tool for stress management.

A Day of Reckoning

We all experience stress every day of our lives. It cannot be avoided in the time-pressured, competitive, and hectic activities of our society. Quiet time has become harder to find as pressure to use every moment of the day productively increases, sometimes consuming our lives. Your body does not recognize the difference between real stress and imagined stress. The physiological response is the same whether you just missed the last bus, which will make you late for an appointment, you were just scared out of your wits by an oncoming car, or you were accosted by a mugger. You are likely to have the same response if you get overlooked for a long-awaited promotion, get in an argument with your spouse over money, or have to stand in line too long at the bank.

When you experience stress from these pressures, your heart rate increases, and your heart beats harder, which in turn increases your blood pressure. Your respiration rate speeds up, you feel a churning in your stomach, and your muscles tense to prepare for action. This state is called hyper-arousal (more commonly known as the fight-or-flight response). All of these reactions are activated by the sympathetic branch of the autonomic nervous system through the release of adrenaline and a multitude of hormones and brain chemicals.

If you are able to physically act out the appropriate response to the event, e.g., run to catch the bus, jump out of the way of the car, or knock out the mugger using your newest karate move, you will use the systems that have been triggered by the fight-or-flight reaction, and the stress will be (at least partially) relieved.

But most of the stressful events in our daily lives are not situations we can resolve by physically acting on them. Most are social and emotional interactions that cause us to feel threatened, angry, embarrassed, or anxious. When we are unable to physically react to them, our bodies internalize the response to the stress, and the physiological chain of events described above gets locked in the body.

The result of that internalization can be chronic high blood pressure, insomnia, headaches, heart palpitations, panic attacks, or chronic anxiety and back pain. Pain and tension in the neck and teeth grinding as well as clinical depression are also often tied to high stress levels. Sustained high levels of stress can bring on any one of the aforementioned disorders, or all of them.

If the internalization continues, and the person suffering from stress does seek out some method of reducing or relieving the negative effects on the body, what follows is the actual breakdown of the body's systems. This can ultimately lead to dysfunction, disease, and even death.

Keeping Body and Soul Together

The key to the relief of internal stress is the parasympathetic branch of the autonomic nervous system. It is the mediator, the soothsayer. It slows down our responses and returns the body to a calm and relaxed state It triggers the *relaxation response,* which counteracts the fight-or-flight response. During the relaxation response, the heart and respiration rates slow down, blood pressure declines, and tension leaves the muscles. Your entire body quiets down.

Slow belly breathing stimulates the parasympathetic nervous system. Nose inhalation, as opposed to mouth inhalation, is also thought to be tied to the parasympathetic system. Inhalation appears to excite the sympathetic nervous system and exhalation the parasympathetic. By inhaling slowly, through your nose, as you do the stretches, breathing rhythmically, and exhaling slowly through your mouth, you will aid your body's ability to relax the muscles and allow them to lengthen.

Research has shown that people who regularly meditate and practice other disciplines that put them into the relaxation response are less susceptible to the fight-or-flight response. By taking a few minutes of quiet, uninterrupted time for belly breathing, followed by these stretches, you will be giving yourself a most precious gift of effective, preventive health care.

The first moving stretch is one that may not be for everyone. If you have chronic instability or pain in the sacro-iliac area or have had a herniated disc, this move may cause you discomfort. That is a signal you should avoid this stretch for now Pain is always a signal from the body that something is not right. If that is the case, move on to the next stretch and listen to your body for feedback.

Some of the stretches involve holding a position after the movement. Hold until you feel your body release into the stretch. If at any time it becomes uncomfortable, return to the starting position.

Note: Remember, the program was designed with the progression of positions from your back, to one side, onto your stomach, onto your hands and knees, and then repeating the progression on the other side. When done that way you will be repeating the stomach and hands and knees stretches twice. This is the most effective way to do the program, but it is also the most time-consuming. If your time is short, after each side-lying stretch, roll over and repeat on the other side.

Exercise 59 Double Bent-Knee Body Rolls with Angels in the Snow

Lie on your back, bend your knees, and place your feet and knees together so that they are touching. Your arms should be in the butterfly stretch, palms up. **Slowly allow both knees to roll to the right** (Illustration 183). Don't force your knees to the right; only release as far as your muscles will let you go. This is a passive move, not an active one. Return to the starting position, then release your knees to the other side. After about eight knee rolls, add the head movement—**as your knees roll right, rotate your head to the right** (Illustration 184). After about four rotations add the arms—**as the legs roll to the right side, slide the left arm along the floor up next to your head and the right arm down to your rolling knees** (Illustrations 185 and 186). Continue to

Illustration 183

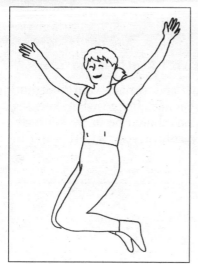

Illustration 184

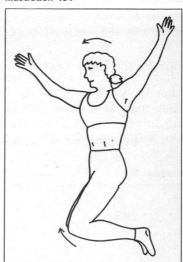

Illustration 185

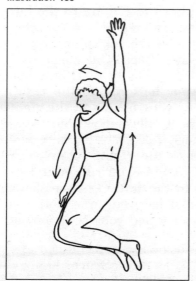

Illustration 186

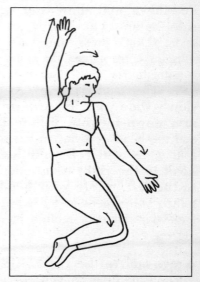

Double-Knee Rolls with Angels in the Snow

slowly roll your knees and head and slide your arms until you feel your range of motion increasing and your body loosening up.

Exercise 60 Single-Knee Roll-ins with Angels in the Snow

Lie on your back, knees bent, and spread your feet and knees apart as wide as they can comfortably go while keeping your feet flat on the floor. Your arms should be in the butterfly stretch (Illustration 187). **Slowly rotate your right knee in**

Illustration 187

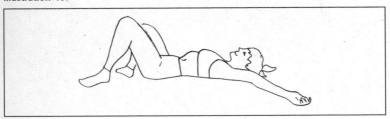

and down, and allow your left knee to fall out to the left side. Return to the starting position and repeat with the other knee. (Don't press your knee in; let the relaxation of your muscles control how far you rotate.) Repeat the single-knee roll-ins to the right and left about eight times (Illustration 188). Then add the arms. **As your legs roll to the right, slowly slide your left arm up by your head and the right arm down by your rolling knees** (Illustration 189). Now, add the head—moving in the same direction as the knees are rolling. **As you roll your legs to the right, rotate your head to the right** (Illustration 190). **As you roll your legs to the left, rotate your head to the left**. Continue slowly rolling your knees and head and sliding your arms until you feel your range of motion increasing and your body loosening up.

✤ *Special Tips*

The key to these two exercises is to keep the motion continuous. Don't pause as you return your legs or head to center.

Illustration 188

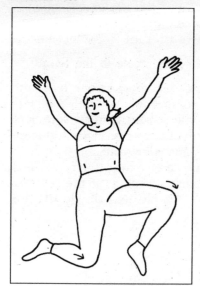

Illustration 189

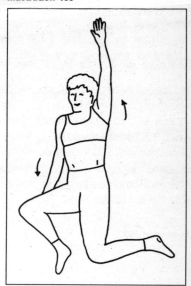

Illustration 190

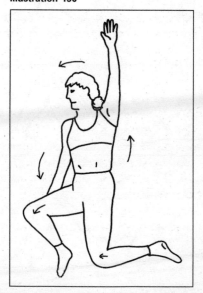

Single-Knee Roll-ins with Angels in the Snow

If the stretch is really feeling great, you *may* pause slightly when you are rotated to the side, but the *rhythmic* motion is what will increase your range of motion the most. Use your breathing by inhaling each time you return to center and exhaling as you roll to the side.

Exercise 61 Supine Pelvic Pump

Lie on your back with your knees bent; spread your feet about 12 inches apart. Let your hands rest on your abdomen (Illustration 191). Inhale deeply and allow the midsection to expand. Exhale slowly and **slowly curl your pelvis toward the ceiling,** feeling the lower back stretch as it presses into the floor (Illustration 192). Inhale deeply, and **slowly tilt the**

Illustration 191

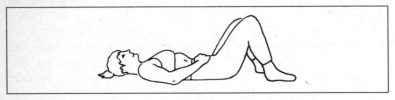

Illustration 192

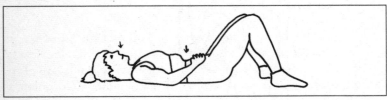

Illustration 193

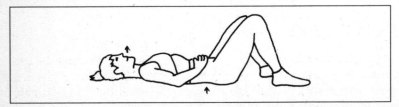

Supine Pelvic Pump

hips into the floor, feeling your lower back lift (Illustration 193). Feel a gentle arching of the entire back. Repeat this slow, continuous pumping motion four to six times. Return to neutral and completely relax.

The next two stretches are wonderful if done slowly. The first one is a stretch you've done several times before; nevertheless, read through the instructions thoroughly before starting each stretch. *Do not jump ahead or skip any steps.* Be sure to stop and allow the back to return to neutral (no tension) between each change in position.

Exercise 62 Double Bent-Knee Body Curl

Lie on your back with your knees bent. Lift your feet off the floor and bring your knees up into a 90-degree angle, holding the outside of your knees with your hands. Allow the legs to open wide to stretch the buttocks. Find "neutral" with your lower back and rest there. Inhale deeply through your nose, and as you exhale, **slowly pull your knees into your chest and gently lift your hips off the floor, keeping the knees apart**. Feel the stretch in your lower back area. **Inhale deeply and as you exhale, slowly tuck your chin and curl your upper body up toward your knees**. Feel the stretch in your upper and midback. **Gently lower your upper body,** keeping your knees pulled to your chest. *Stop and allow the back to relax.* **Slowly lower the hips to the floor, but keep hold of your knees.** Find "neutral" with your back. **Slowly lower your feet to the floor and allow your back to relax.** Extend your legs over your rolled towel or pillow. Completely relax and belly-breathe.

Repeat 1 time.

Exercise 63 Back-Lying Hip Stretch

Lie on your back with your knees bent, your arms in the butterfly position with the *palms down.* Cross the right leg over the left leg and let it relax (Illustration 194). Inhale deeply through your nose, and as you exhale through your mouth **very slowly let the knees to roll to the right** (Illus-

Illustration 194

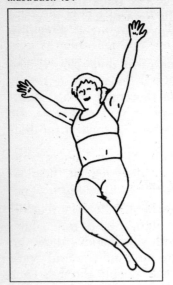

Illustration 195

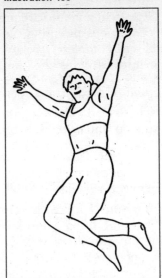

Illustration 196

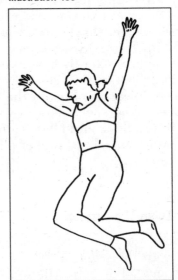

Back-Lying Hip Stretch

tration 195). Keep breathing and **slowly release into the stretch. Now rotate your head to the right** Feel the body opening up (Illustration 196). Hold for a moment, breathing deeply, then slowly return to starting position, uncross your legs, and rest in your bent-knee position. Repeat on the other side.

Repeat 1 or 2 times each side.

Exercise 64 Single Knee to Chest

Lie on your back with your knees bent, your hands resting on your abdomen. Fully extend your right leg on the floor and allow it to relax (Illustration 197). Without lifting your upper body, **lift your left leg and hold your knee in your hands.** Inhale deeply through your nose, and as you exhale through your mouth draw your left leg in to your chest, releasing the lower back (Illustration 198). Return your left foot to the floor and your right leg into the bent-knee starting position. Repeat on the other side.

Repeat 1 or 2 times each side.

Illustration 197

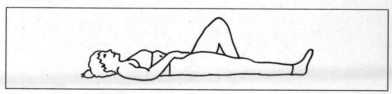

Illustration 198

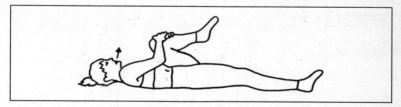

Single Knee to Chest

Exercise 65 Side-Lying Pelvic Pump

Lie on your right side with your head on a pillow or resting on your curled bottom arm. Bend your knees into a fetal position (Illustration 199). Inhale deeply, allowing the midsection to expand, and **slowly rotate your buttocks backward.** Feel your back gently arch (Illustration 200). Exhale slowly, pulling your abdominal wall in and curl your pelvis up toward your chest, feeling your back round (Illustration 201). Repeat

Illustration 199

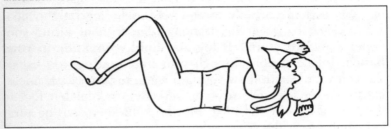

Illustration 200

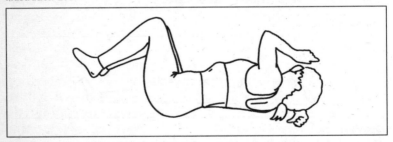

Illustration 201

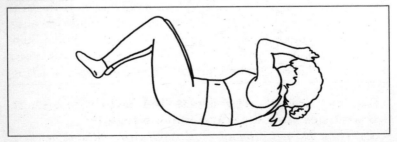

Side-Lying Pelvic Pump

this pumping motion four to six times. Come back to neutral and completely relax.

Exercise 66 Side-Lying Upper Back and Chest Stretch

Lie on your right side with your head on a pillow or resting on your curled bottom arm. Bend your knees into a fetal position. Stretch your arms straight out from the chest perpendicular to the body, palms together (Illustration 202). Keeping your left arm straight, inhale deeply through your nose, and as you exhale through your mouth, **slide your left arm forward as far as you can go, reaching beyond the right hand and then along the floor.** Slightly tuck your chin and allow your head to roll forward as the arm slides (Illustration 203). Breathe deeply through your nose. Keeping your palm on the floor, slide your arm toward your head in an arc as far as you can comfortably go and hold for a count of four (Illustration 204). Feel the stretch all down the side of the arm and back. **Return your arm to its starting position and then slide it back as far as it can go and still have the arm remain straight** (Illustration 205). *Don't allow the upper body to roll backward; the movement is limited to the shoulder blade of your right arm.* Breathing slowly and deeply, slowly repeat the sliding motion four times, inhaling as you slide back, exhaling as you slide forward. **Return to the starting position with your palms together. Slowly lift your left arm up so its fingers are pointed toward the ceiling** (Illustration 206). Inhale deeply. As you exhale, **slowly let the arm fall in back of you, keeping the palm facing up.** Allow your upper body and head to roll backward as the arm lowers, but let your arm lead (Illustration 207). Only lower as far as feels safe and comfortable. Hold until you feel fully stretched, **bend your elbow, place your palm on your chest** (Illustration 208), **and roll back to the starting position.**

Repeat 1 time, then proceed to the next stretch. These two stretches should always be done together.

WARNING: Do not attempt to lift your arm without bending your elbow first.

Illustration 202

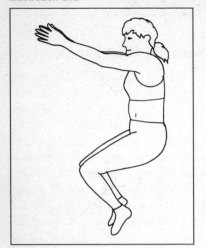

Illustration 203

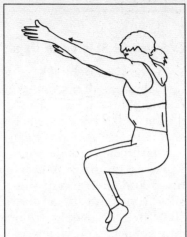

Illustration 204

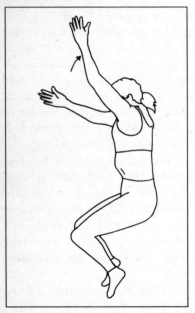

Illustration 205

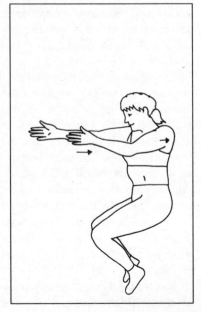

Illustration 206

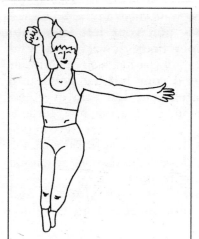

Illustration 207

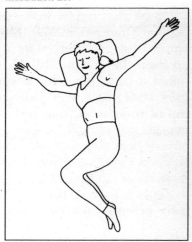

Illustration 208

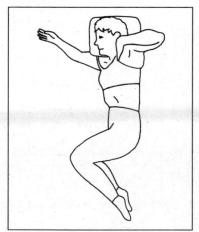

Side-Lying Upper Back and Chest Stretch

Exercise 67 Side-Lying Curl and Extension

Lie on your right side, keeping your knees in the 90-degree position (Illustration 209). **Slowly pull your left knee into your chest and curl your upper body down into a fetal position** (Illustration 210). Hold until you feel a stretch in your rounded back, then **slowly extend your left leg down and fully straighten it as you stretch your left arm over the top of your head.** Your body should be in a long line (Illustration 211). Your right, supporting knee stays bent as the top side of your body stretches out fully. Hold until you feel the stretch all down the front of your body. Repeat the curl and extension three times. Return to the starting position.

Repeat 1 time, then roll over onto your stomach and fully extend your body with your forehead on the floor

Illustration 209   **Illustration 210**   **Illustration 211**

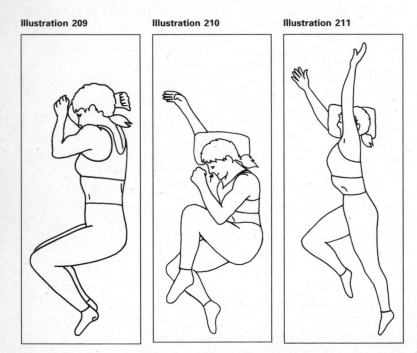

Side-Lying Curl and Extension

and your arms over your head. Allow your body to completely relax. If you are not continuing the rest of the
stretches at this time, roll over and repeat on the
other side.

Exercise 68 Prone Diagonal Extension

Lie on the floor on your stomach with your arms extended
above your head, palms down (Illustration 212). Inhale deeply
through your nose, and as you exhale through your mouth,
**pull your abdominals in and up and lift your right leg
off the floor about 2 inches and hold** (Illustration 213).
Keep your forehead on the floor and **lift your left arm about
2 inches** (Illustration 214). Stretch diagonally from your fingertips to your toes, then **slowly lower your arm and leg
to the floor** and completely relax. Pull your abdominals in
and up and repeat with the other arm and leg.
    Repeat 1 time.

Illustration 212

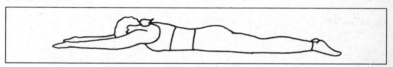

Illustration 213

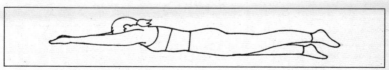

Illustration 214

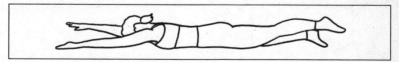

Prone Diagonal Extension

Exercise 69 Cat Back Stretch Combo

First, you may want to refer to Exercise 51, on page 177, for illustrated positions. Get on your hands and knees with your arms directly under your shoulders and your knees a comfortable distance apart. **Tuck your chin and pelvis and fully round your back** (Illustration 158). Hold long enough to feel the muscles stretch. **Gently push your rib cage out to the right and hold** (see Illustration 159), **then to the left** (see Illustration 160). **Slowly lower your back, raise your chin, and extend your buttocks out in back, allowing the middle of your back to gently drop into a "sagging bridge"** (see Illustration 161). Feel your shoulder blades move together. *Spread your knees wide apart* (your toes will be closer together), and **slowly lower yourself back onto your heels** (Illustration 215). **Place your forehead on the floor and stretch your arms out in front of you as far as you can** (palms down) in what I call the prayer position (Illustration 216). Hold until you feel the stretch down the

Illustration 215

Illustration 216

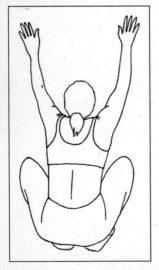

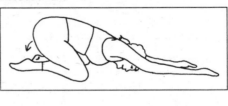

Cat Back Stretch Combo (*top view*)

sides of your back and in the inner thigh and groin area, then stay in position 219 and begin the next stretch (see Illustration 217).

The next stretch should immediately follow this one. If you are not able to sit back on your heels, or if that portion of the stretch stresses your back, do only the cat back and sagging bridge. If you can sit back, this is a great stretch for the inner thigh.

♣ *Special Tips*

Use your breathing throughout this stretch, inhaling deeply through your nose before you begin each movement, and exhaling slowly as you actually do the move. Breathe easily through your nose as you hold the position.

Exercise 70 Prayer Position Back and Chest Stretch

Assume the prayer position—draw your left arm back close to your chest, bending at the elbow, and rest your forehead on the back of your left hand (Illustration 217). Stretch your right arm diagonally forward, keeping your palm on the floor,

Illustration 217   **Illustration 218**   **Illustration 219**

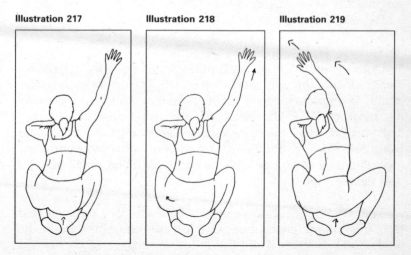

Prayer Position Back and Chest Stretch (*top view*)

and allow your hips to come up off your heels (Illustration 218). Hold until you *feel* the stretch in your chest, arm, and all down the side of your body. **Slowly slide your right arm over to the left,** still stretching forward, **to increase the stretch** (Illustration 219). Move slowly back to the starting position. Repeat with other arm.

Repeat 1 time. The next stretch should immediately follow this one.

Exercise 71 Extended Abdominal and Hip Flexor Stretch

Starting from the prayer position (Illustration 220), **push back up onto your hands and knees. Walk yourself forward on your hands until the tops of your knees are touching the floor.** Turn your toes slightly out, allowing your pelvic area to open. Keep your elbows straight to raise your upper body a little higher. Keep your neck relaxed and in line with your spine (Illustration 221). **Gently stretch your chin forward.** Hold until you feel the stretch in your abdomen and down the front of your body. You may feel a tightening in your lower back. Hold only as long as is comfortable, then **slowly walk your hands back to the prayer position** (Illustration 222). Completely relax.

Repeat 1 time.

❖ *Special Tips*

Once again, use your breathing throughout this stretch, inhaling deeply through your nose before you begin each movement, and exhaling slowly through your mouth as you actually do the move. Breathe easily through your nose as you hold the position. If you have only done the side-lying exercises on your left side, at this point you should roll onto your right side and repeat exercises 65 through 72. Then continue with the next stretch.

This stretch is also a great strengthener. It is complex and requires intense concentration. I use the same exercise in the abdominal program. Here the focus is on the stretch, not the pulling in and up of the abdominals. Read the instructions

Illustration 220

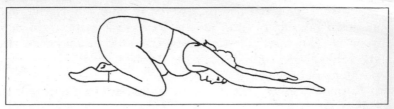

Illustration 221

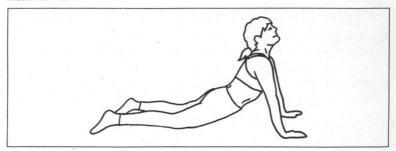

Illustration 222

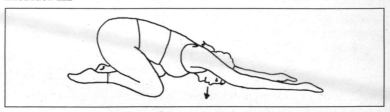

Extended Abdominal and Hip Flexor Stretch

thoroughly before trying it, and take note of the small details. They are all important.

Exercise 72 Hands and Knees Diagonal Extension

Get on your hands and knees. Move your knees directly under your hips and your arms directly under your shoulders (Illustration 223). Your pelvis and rib cage should be level. Inhale deeply through your nose, and as you exhale through

Illustration 223

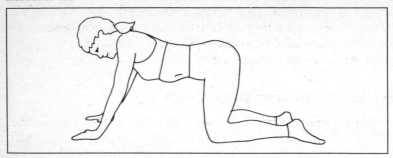

Illustration 224

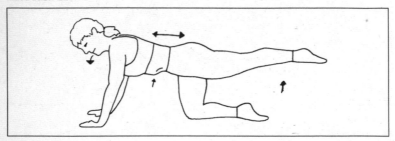

Illustration 225

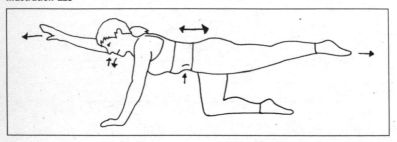

Hands and Knees Diagonal Extension

your mouth, gently pull your abdominals in and up. **Slowly slide your left leg back until it is fully extended. Keep your toes on the floor. Slowly lift your left leg until it is in a direct line with your back** (Illustration 224). **Slowly lift your right arm out in front of you until it too is in a direct line with your back.** *Do not raise your chin.* Keep your head and neck in line with your back (Illustration 225). Hold for a count of four and breathe. Slowly lower your arm. Slowly lower your leg until your toes touch the floor, and return to the starting position. Sit back and relax.

Repeat on the other side.

Exercise 73 Lowering Bridge Stretch

Lie on your back with your knees bent, feet flat on the floor. Slide your arms down next to your hips into a V. **Contract your buttocks and raise your body up onto the back of your shoulder blades into a bridge** (Illustration 226). **Slowly lower your body, curling your pelvis up. Turn your palms up and slide your arms up next to your head as you lift your toes up** (Illustration 227). Heels stay on the floor. Allow your lower back to gently arch up off the floor. Repeat this combination of movements several times. Return to the starting position and rest.

Illustration 226

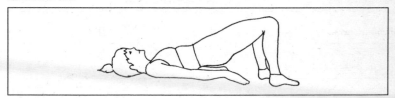

Illustration 227

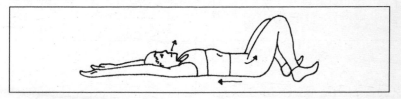

Lowering Bridge Stretch

❖ *Special Tips*

Time your breathing throughout this stretch so that you are inhaling as you lift up and exhaling as you lower your body.

Exercise 74 Single Knee-to-Chest Curl and Extension

Lie on your back with your knees bent, feet flat on the floor. Slide your left leg out until it is fully extended. Lift your right leg up. Hold your right knee with both your hands and allow your body to completely relax (Illustration 228). Inhale deeply, then **slowly exhale as you pull your knee to your chest. Tuck your chin and curl your upper body toward the outside of your right knee** (Illustration 229). Inhaling deeply, **slowly lower your upper body and extend your right leg straight up.** Feel the stretch in the back of the leg and the buttocks (Illustration 230). Repeat the upper body curl, **this time drawing your upper body to the inside of your right knee** (Illustration 231). Alternate this move two more times, alternating first to the outside and then to the inside of your knee. Slowly release and place your right foot flat on the floor with your knee bent and allow your body to completely relax.

Repeat with the other leg.

Illustration 228

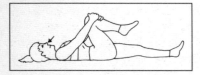

Illustration 229

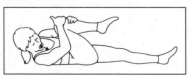

Illustration 230

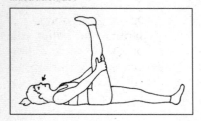

Illustration 231

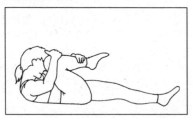

Single Knee-to-Chest Curl and Extension

Exercise 75 Full Supine Starfish Extension

Lie on your back with your legs fully extended, arms in the butterfly position, with palms facing up (Illustration 232). Inhale deeply and fully. As you exhale, **slowly slide your legs out into a V as you slide your arms down toward your hips. Gently curl your pelvis up** (Illustration 233). Then inhale deeply again and **slowly slide your legs together as you slide your arms up over your head** (Illustration 234). Stretch your body out from each fingertip to your toes. Feel the stretch in your arms, legs, abdomen, and back. Slowly exhale and repeat the sequence several more times. When you feel completely stretched and relaxed, *stop* wherever you are in the sequence. Notice what you feel.

You have just completed seventeen stretches that should have thoroughly loosened your entire body. These stretches don't require the highly structured body positions of the abdominal and back-strengthening exercises. They are meant to be adapted to the individual by modifying *your* body position to fit the stretch. Alter any of the positions or directions that are necessary to make the stretch feel good! For instance, if having your knees wide apart in the prayer position is uncomfortable, keep your knees together. If curling your pelvis up during the Starfish Extension doesn't feel good, do the stretch without! *Don't do any stretch that causes you to feel pain.* It's important that these stretches feel good and are pleasurable; otherwise, you won't do them.

Stretch tension is uncomfortable, and you will probably feel some of that when you first start the program, but you should not feel pain. If you do, it means the stretch may not be for you.

Take a minute and *listen* to your body. Where and how does it want to move? Adjust your position and try the stretch again. If you still experience discomfort, don't try it again. Go on to the next stretch. The key to making these stretches safe and effective for your body is *moving slowly*. That means finding a rhythm that is gentle and fluid and allows you to stay relaxed while you perform the stretch. Fast movement requires muscle tension. Slowly exhaling as you move in the direction of the stretch, and breathing deeply as you hold any position, will maximize your release into it.

Illustration 232

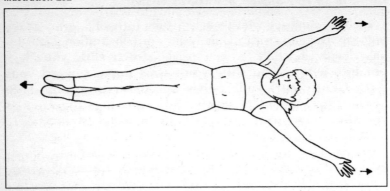

Illustration 233

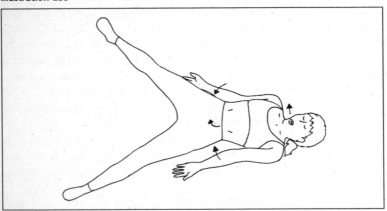

Illustration 234

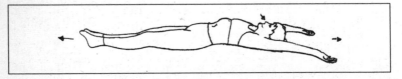

Full Supine Starfish Extension

Put on soothing music to help set the mood, turn the telephone off, ask family members not to disturb you, and plan your stretch time just before or after a warm bath or shower. All will help you relax and fully experience the benefits of these stretches.

Our bodies are miraculous machines that we usually take for granted until something goes wrong. Give your body the gift of your undivided attention for just a few minutes each day and see how your whole attitude (as well as your physical well-being) improves.

Remember, just as with all the other parts of this program, it is not necessary to do all the stretches. Try them at least once, then pick out the ones that you like best and do them after your back-strengthening exercises. Choose one or two to do in the morning before you get out of bed or just before you go to sleep at night. If you have the time to pamper yourself, do the whole stretching program, start to finish. It will take you about 30 minutes. You won't believe how good you will feel. You deserve it!

Doing Your Own Thing

If you want a totally different experience, but one that achieves the same improved flexibility, try free-style stretching.

This is completely unstructured and can take anywhere from 5 to 15 minutes, depending on how much you are enjoying it. For many in my relaxation classes it becomes a kind of moving meditation.

Find a private place where you can be totally uninhibited. Put on some music, something sensual and with a slow rhythmic beat, like jazz. I also like to use African and Caribbean music. I suggest that you start in one of three positions—on your hands and knees, lying on your back, or lying on your side. You want to feel supported, balanced, stable, and comfortable.

Close your eyes. (This *is* a requirement.) Listen to the music for a minute, then begin to move any way you feel inclined. You might start by gently swaying from side to side, or rocking if you are lying on the floor. Then try rolling. Up, down, around—any direction that feels good to your body.

Tuck your chin, round your back, stick your butt out, roll your shoulders. Do what comes naturally, and let yourself go. When you're tired of that, change positions. Roll around, rock around, undulate. Imagine your body is made entirely of water and move without restrictions or a controlled direction. Express yourself. You can use elements from the structured stretches and roll them together in any order you want.

This isn't as weird as it sounds. Loosen up and give it a try. No one can see you—you've found a private place to experiment, right? But do it, because it is the most free form of stretching you will ever do and it works.

I began free-style stretching with my Senior Exercise class some time ago. At first the women were inhibited and uncomfortable letting their bodies go. Now, they tell me they do it at home, on their own, because it makes them feel s-o-o-o good.

9

Standing Up for Yourself

I've devoted quite a few pages to persuading you of the value of moving stretches because too few people take advantage of them. That's not to diminish the role static stretches play in maintaining a healthy, balanced musculoskeletal system. Static stretches are essential for muscles that have been exercised at a fairly intense level for a sustained period of time. Whether you power walk (my personal favorite), run, cycle, ride a mountain bike, work out on a stair climber, or take aerobics classes, static stretches are the recommended physical chaser.

For many years, we were told to stretch before beginning to exercise. Now we understand that static stretching of cold muscles results in damage to the muscle tissue and can cause injury. We have replaced preexertion stretching with *warming up*.

A good warm-up prevents muscle strains and tears by gradually increasing the core temperature of the muscles, increasing the flow of oxygen and fluids through muscle tissues and initiating the first lengthening of the muscle fibers before we begin more strenuous exercise.

Prolonged exercise results in accumulated tension in the muscle fibers, buildup of toxic waste products within the muscles, and microscopic tears in the muscle tissue. These stresses cause a chemical reaction (a release of new proteins) that results in a buildup or increase in size of the muscle fibers

called *hypertrophy,* which is the process that causes muscles
to get bigger and stronger. It will occur if appropriate attention is paid to care of the body in other ways—e.g., adequate
nutrition, stretching, rest, and so forth. It is the desired result
for a body builder or anyone else wanting to increase the size
and definition of his or her muscles.

Pulling Yourself Together

Delayed Onset Muscle Soreness, often called DOMS, is believed to be a result of eccentric muscle contractions. The
words *eccentric contraction* describe the action in a muscle
lengthened against resistance, as when you are lowering a
heavy weight. When the muscle shortens to perform work,
lifting a heavy weight, that's called a *concentric* muscle contraction. I explained earlier that muscles shorten as their fibers
slide or telescope into each other. Well, because the fibers
are designed to contract, the muscles aren't really stressed
unless you are trying to lift an unreasonable amount of weight.
Even then, the stress is not on the muscle itself, but on the
muscle-tendinous junction, where the tendon attaches to the
bone.

On the other hand, when you lengthen a muscle, the muscle
fibers and connective tissues that bind the muscle together
experience stress. Microscopic tearing and a breakdown of the
contractile elements occur. This results in chemical changes
within the muscle that produce inflammation and soreness.
Static stretching is appropriate *after* strenuous exercise, because it increases the blood flow to the fatigued and stressed
tissues, flushes toxic waste from the cells, and begins the process of recovery for the muscle tissues.

Unfortunately, static stretching has been seriously misused.
People simply stretch all their muscles, *whether they need to
or not,* and contribute to the muscle imbalances already present in their bodies. If you sit at a desk all day and know your
hamstrings are tight because you can't straighten your legs all
the way out, you may not need to stretch the front of your
thighs, just the back. If you have a job where you stand all
day (most likely with your knees locked back), don't stretch

your hamstrings, just stretch your quadriceps. As you begin to feel positive changes after a few weeks of targeted stretching, you can begin to stretch all the muscles in your legs. By the way, almost everyone can benefit by stretching their calf muscles. All weight-bearing motion uses the muscles in the lower legs and the feet, so stretching this area every day (after some activity) is a good idea.

The following are a few simple, common static stretches for the calf muscles, the hamstrings, and the quadriceps. I've also included a few for the upper body. The leg stretches are more effective if you are able to do them against a ledge, such as a step, block of wood, or even a curb. If none of these things are handy, you can do the exercises against a wall. Remember that all these stretches should *follow* some form of activity. Hold each stretch for a slow count of thirty, and always release slowly. If you sit with your upper back rounded all day, you may not *need* to stretch your upper back. Concentrate on the stretches for the chest and front of the shoulder, lower back, and sides.

Exercise 76 Standing Calf Stretch

Stand facing a step or block of wood. Put your right foot in front of you and the ball of your foot against the step. Pull your abdominals in and up, lengthen your spine, and keep your chest lifted. **Holding on to something for support** (the back of a chair or a railing), **rise onto the toe of your left foot and press forward so that your right foot bends at the ankle and at the toes** (Illustration 235). Feel the stretch down the back of the right leg. Slowly count to twenty. **Slightly bend your right knee and press into the top of your foot** (Illustration 236). You will feel the stretch move into your ankle. Hold for a slow count of ten. Release and repeat with legs in reversed position.

Illustration 235

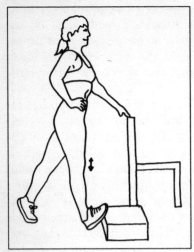

Illustration 236

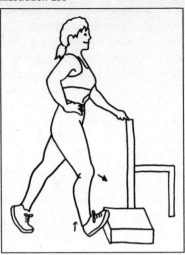

Standing Calf Stretch

Exercise 77 Standing Hamstring Stretch

Stand facing a raised surface such as a stair, bench, chair, or low table. It should be about 12 inches high (adjust for your height and physical condition). You may support yourself by holding on to the back of a chair on the stair rail. **Place your right heel on the top of the stair or bench, with your toes pointed up.** Make sure the foot you are standing on is facing front, not turned out. Keep the knee of your standing leg slightly bent. Inhale deeply through your nose and exhale slowly as you begin the stretch. **Lean forward from the hip, bringing your chest forward, not down** (Illustration 237). You should feel the stretch in the buttock and back of your leg, not in your low back. Let the leg lengthen in this position for a count of twenty. Now, gently contract the front of your right thigh, and hold for a count of ten. Release the contraction in your thigh and move your chest forward just a little more. Feel the increased stretch. Lower your leg and repeat with the other side.

Illustration 237

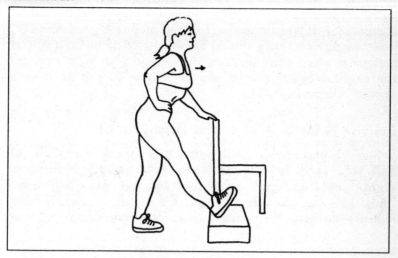

Standing Hamstring Stretch

Illustration 238

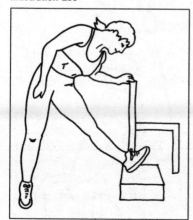

Illustration 239

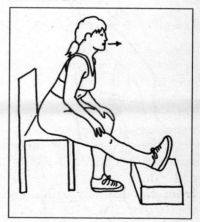

Special Tips for Exercise 77

❖ *Special Tips*

Make sure you keep your chest lifted and forward as you stretch; do not let it drop or round your upper back. Keep your spine as erect as you can. If you want to stretch your inner thigh, at the end of the stretch, rotate your left foot out to 90 degrees and gently bend over your stretched leg (Illustration 238). If you are unable to stand on one leg comfortably, you may stretch sitting down. Place your chair in front of the surface you are using to stretch on. Place your right heel on the surface. Inhale deeply and begin the stretch as written above (Illustration 239).

Exercise 78 Standing Quadriceps (Thigh) Stretch

Stand supporting yourself with a stair railing or chair back. **Lift your right heel behind you, hold your foot in your right hand, and pull your foot toward your buttocks.** Make sure the knee on your left leg is soft or slightly bent (Illustration 240). Keep your legs as close together as you can

Illustration 240

Illustration 241

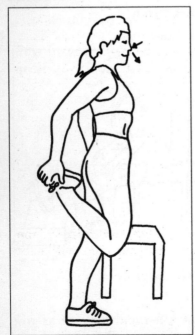
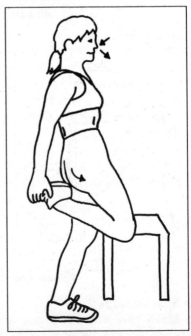

Standing Quadriceps (Thigh) Stretch

during the stretch. Pull your abdominals in and up and lengthen your spine as you hold for a slow count of twenty. Staying in the same position, **contract your buttocks and tilt your pelvis forward and hold for a slow count of ten** (Illustration 241). Release and repeat with the left leg.

✤ *Special Tip*

If you are unable to stand on one leg you may also do this stretch seated. If you are unable to pull your foot toward your buttocks, you may simply bend your knee and place the top of your foot on a chair seat or low table and then complete the stretch as written above.

Exercise 79 Standing Upper Back Stretch

Stand with your legs shoulder width apart, and your knees soft or slightly bent. Pull your abdominals in and up and raise your arms in front of you, chest high. Interlace your fingers with the palms facing you. Inhale deeply and as you exhale, slowly drop your chin onto your chest and pull forward with your arms, rounding your upper back (Illustration 242). Keep your lower back in neutral and the tops of your shoulders relaxed. Breathe normally for a count of five and inhale deeply through your nose, and as you exhale through your mouth, gently rotate your arms to the left and hold for a count of ten, breathing easily (Illustration 243). Inhale deeply and slowly rotate to the right as you exhale (Illustration 244). Hold and breathe normally for a count of ten. Release.

✤ *Special Tips*

You may do this stretch seated. Sit near the edge of the seat, with your feet flat on the floor and your hips and knees at right angles (Illustration 245).

Illustration 242

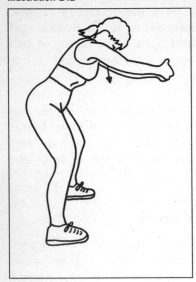

Illustration 243

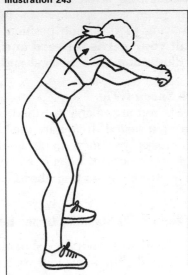

Illustration 244

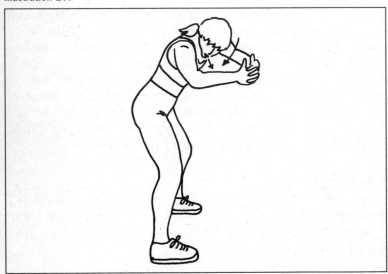

Standing Upper Back Stretch

Illustration 245

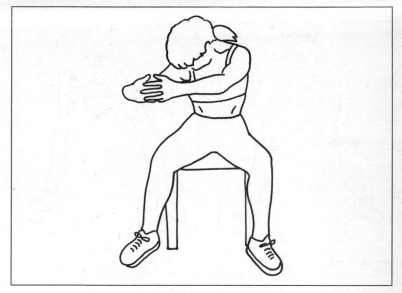

Special Tips for Exercise 79

Exercise 80 Standing Buttock and Back Stretch

Stand with your legs wide apart and bend your knees. Bend forward, supporting yourself with your hands on your thighs. Let your buttocks extend out in back of you (Illustration 246). Inhale deeply and exhale slowly as you begin the stretch. **Press your right shoulder forward and down as you gently rotate and look over your left shoulder** (Illustration 247). Your right arm should remain straight; your left may bend (Illustration 248). Breathe normally while you hold for a count of ten. Keep your neck relaxed. Return to your starting position. Inhale deeply and then exhale slowly as you rotate and repeat with your left shoulder. You should feel this stretch all down the side of your body.

Illustration 246

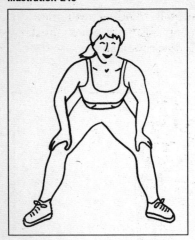

Illustration 247

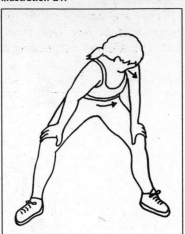

Illustration 248

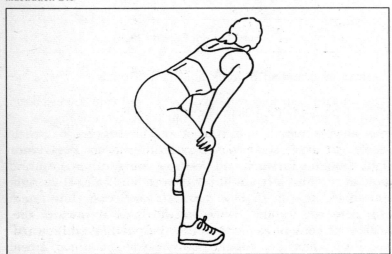

Standing Buttock and Back Stretch

✤ *Special Tips*

If you are unable to do this stretch standing, you may do it seated. Make sure you sit with your legs wide apart (Illustration 249). Follow the instructions as written above.

Illustration 249

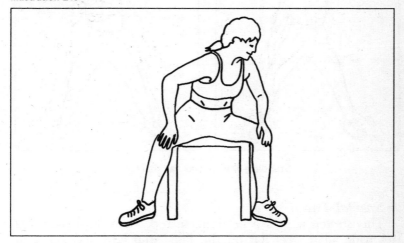

Special Tips for Exercise 80

Exercise 81 Standing Tricep and Lat Stretch

Stand with your legs shoulder- or hip- width apart. **Raise your right arm and bend it at the elbow to drop your hand behind your head.** Your elbow will be pointing toward the ceiling (Illustration 250). **Pull your abdominals in and up. Inhale deeply as you reach up with your left hand and grab your right elbow. Gently pull it toward the midline of your body as you exhale slowly. Bend forward from the waist very slightly and hold for a count of ten** (Illustration 251). You should feel this all down the side of your body into the top of your hip. Release and repeat with the other side.

Illustration 250

Illustration 251

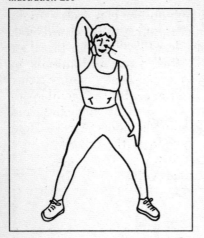 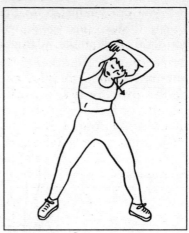

Standing Tricep and Lat Stretch

✤ *Special Tips*

This stretch may also be done seated. Make sure your legs are wide apart, feet flat on the floor, and hips and knees at right angles (Illustration 252).

Illustration 252

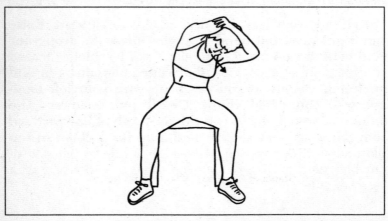

Special Tips for Exercise 81

Exercise 82 Standing Chest and Shoulder Stretch

Postion yourself next to a door frame or two walls at right angles. Raise your right arm with your palm forward and, bending your elbow, place your hand flat against the door frame or wall (Illustration 253). **Pull your abdominals in and up. Inhale deeply, and as you exhale, rotate your body slowly away from your bent arm.** Be very gentle with this move, feeling the stretch in the front of your chest and shoulder (Illustration 254). Keep your shoulders relaxed. Hold for a count of ten. Release and repeat on the other side.

Illustration 253

Illustration 254

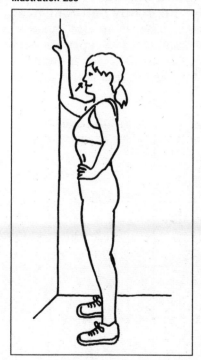
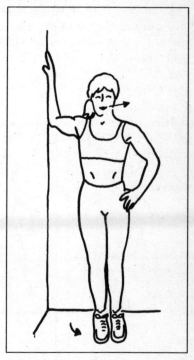

Standing Chest and Shoulder Stretch

✤ *Special Tips*

This is harder to do sitting, but if you need to, place your chair where you would stand and sit on the edge of the seat with your legs apart and your feet flat on the floor.

Exercise 83 Standing or Seated Neck Stretch

Stand with your legs shoulder width apart (Illustration 255) or sit in a chair with your feet flat on the floor and your hips and knees at right angles. Allow both arms to hang straight down by your side. Your head should be centered over your spine with your neck relaxed. **Inhale deeply as you reach up with your left hand and place it on your right temple** (Illustration 256). **Exhale slowly and gently pull your head over toward your left shoulder.** *Keep your face centered; do not rotate your head* (Illustration 257). Keep your neck and shoulders relaxed and breathe normally for a count of ten. Very slowly return to the starting position and repeat on the other side.

Illustration 255   **Illustration 256**   **Illustration 257**

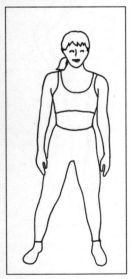
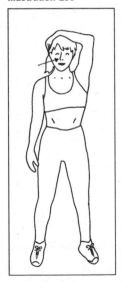
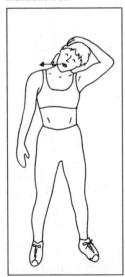

Standing or Seated Neck Stretch

There you have it. A complete static stretching program. No matter what your condition, there is something for you in this program. Modifying is the name of the game. If a stretch doesn't feel quite right (but doesn't hurt), try adjusting your body position slightly or do it seated. If you give your body the attention it deserves, it will tell you what it wants and needs.

Now go on to the last chapter, where I will tell you some other ways to incorporate these exercises into your life.

10

Wrapping It Up

Are you ready to incorporate all these new movements into your daily life? My main objective in developing these exercises and stretches was to make them easy to do and effective. The most effective exercise program in the world does you no good if you don't follow it. Often people don't follow their exercise programs because it's too difficult to get to the gym, or if they *do* have the time, they discover that they forgot to bring their workout clothes, or the weather is bad, or they only have fifteen minutes—obviously not enough time to exercise! The President's Council on Physical Fitness reports that obstacles of this sort keep 80 percent of the population from exercising regularly. The most common reason people give is "not enough time."

You can be different. You have at your fingertips (literally) a whole new approach to strengthening. Granted, this book addresses only abdominal and back strengthening, but let my approach permeate your whole concept of exercise. Find a way to integrate it into your life.

This is an exercise program for real people. People with busy schedules and families. People who may have more than just essential body fat. People with back pain. The abdominal exercises were not designed to give you a rippling outer abdominal wall. They were designed to give you strong, firm, *deep* abdominals that provide support for your back and improve your posture and functional body mechanics. They will dramatically change the way you look. Your newly strengthened internal corset will lift and support your ribs, decompress your lumbar spine, and hold in your abdomen, thereby relieving the pull and strain on your lower back. They will create a leaner, pulled-in look and accentuate your waist. Every one of my clients who has been consistent about the exercises has a measurably smaller waistline—though they haven't lost any weight at all.

Flat as a Pancake

Let me spell out exactly what this program can and can't do. It will not take fat off of your belly or "spot reduce." What it does is make the deep abdominal wall tighter, giving it more tone. This automatically pulls the belly in, and fat pulled in looks better than fat that sticks out.

As we get older our bodies increase the amount of fat storage from the foods we eat. This is for a variety of reasons. As we age, our production of lean muscle mass decreases. Although the reasons aren't thoroughly understood, research has shown that there is a 3 to 5 percent loss of muscle tissue every decade after the age of 25.

Hormonal changes and a slowing down of the metabolism are responsible for a lot of this. Our sedentary lifestyles also play a role. Children are always on the move. Adults tend to sit most of the day. As we get older our bodies rely more on carbohydrates for fuel than on fat. Therefore, it takes more activity to burn fat as you get older, not less. Less activity uses less lean muscle mass, so we lose it (it's the old "use it or lose it" cliché). The more muscle mass we lose, the fewer calories we burn. It's a vicious cycle.

Yes, you can gain body fat even if your body weight has not increased. So don't be surprised about your body changing shape even though you haven't gained any weight. Not only does our production of body fat increase, but the places we store fat on our bodies also shift. As our hormone levels change, fat begins to collect around our bellies, in both men and women. Women may lose the curvaceous hips and thighs they had when they were in their twenties or thirties, and they're left with extra weight on the upper hip and lower abdominal area. Men often lose their muscular chests, arms, and legs, and develop a loose roll of fat directly around their middle.

I'm not telling you this to discourage you, but to make you aware that our body shapes are going to change (or maybe already have), and that even these extraordinary exercises cannot give you back your twenty-five-year-old body or guarantee you a totally flat abdomen.

As I said before, most of these unwelcome changes are actually caused by a decrease in physical activity, combined with poor eating habits. It is the lack of exercise—consistent, daily physical activity—that causes us to lose muscle tone. It is the overconsumption of fats, foods inadequate nutrition, and alcohol in our diets that creates the roll of fat on our bellies.

The good news is that these changes can be controlled and even reversed with strength training and aerobic exercise such as walking.

Picture of Health

Now that you have begun this new approach to caring for your body, I hope you support it with other behaviors and habits that will enhance the "new you."

That means getting some form of aerobic exercise, for at least twenty or thirty minutes several times a week, preferably every day. That aerobic exercise may consist of walking at a pace brisk enough to increase your heart and respiratory rate, riding a bicycle, or any other moderate activity that you sustain for at least twenty minutes.

It also means eating a healthy diet. By healthy I mean one that is low in fat, well balanced, and high in nutritional content. You need to provide fuel for your body to make all these positive changes. Taking care of yourself also means making the time to be with yourself and allowing your mind to quiet. These exercises are the ideal way to do just that.

If you don't know how or where to start your new health and self-care habits, call your local hospital and ask for its health promotions or wellness department and ask the staff there to recommend local personal trainers and nutritional counselors. *If you feel at all unsure about what you're doing, get assistance.* That's what those departments are for. They'll love it if you call!

If you already do some form of regular exercise or sport, notice how being in your body in this new way enhances your performance. You should feel stronger, more stable, and better balanced, and have more energy.

If there is a Yoga or T'ai Chi class offered near you, I suggest that you try them. They are wonderful ways to get in touch with your body, while offering very effective, gentle strengthening for your muscles.

Practice Makes Perfect

In the beginning it is important to be religious in your daily practice of these exercises. The more you practice, the faster you'll see results. Our lives are not predictable; that's what makes it so difficult to adhere to programs with specific requirements. The only requirement for this program is that you be open to new ideas about strengthening and be willing to improve your total well-being, physically, mentally, and spiritually.

Because you can do the in and up move in virtually every body position there is (though I admit I haven't tried it standing on my head!), you can do the exercises *all day long*. In chapter 1 I talked about fitting the exercises into your daily life. Because this program builds functional strength, you will begin to use the new, strengthening moves in your everyday activities.

Focus on pulling **in and up** tightly every time you climb stairs. If you are listening to music on the radio, at home, at work, or in your car, pull in and up tightly for the length of one whole song. If you are standing in line at the grocery store or at the bank, practice pulling in and up until you get to the counter. See if you can do it and stay relaxed enough to complete your purchase, and (of course) still breathe.

It is important to do the exercises in the various positions suggested, because in real life we vary our body positions all day long. Each position offers a different level and form of resistance. Although almost everyone tells me that within a week they are practicing the move while they are driving, this is probably the least effective variation of all. When you are sitting, your pelvis is passively rotated, shortening the muscles in the lower abdomen. This means that the abdominal muscles can't contract any farther. The muscle fibers may shorten a little, but they have very little to lift or pull, so there is no resistance.

The exercises are most effective when you are in a weight-bearing position (on your feet), which is when our lower backs need the most support. That's why doing the basic in and up move all through the day, whenever you are on your feet, is important. When I am power walking or running, I do a form of active in and up that allows me to breathe deeper and harder than normal, and I'm strengthening my abdominals in an intense way. Using the in and up move when you are swimming enables you to hold your body higher in the water (you'll move faster and more smoothly).

If you live in snow country (as I do), use the *in and up* move (I call it "putting the corset on") every time you are shoveling snow. It will save your back. When you are mopping the floor or doing laundry or ironing, "put the corset on." When you are working in the garden, raking leaves, or working on your car, "put the corset on." If you are horseback riding, wind surfing, or skiing, "put the corset on." In every one of these activities, having the corset on increases your stability. It allows you to move as a unit—strong, flexible, and well supported.

Your performance in the pivotal sports such as golf and tennis is also greatly enhanced by the corset, but these sports require you to be completely relaxed as you hold your abdominals in and up. It takes more practice and will become easier to relax after you have done the program for several months.

If you've suffered from chronic back pain, this program will come as a wonderful surprise. These exercises and stretches will actually make a difference in your life. The key is to select both abdominal exercises and the stretches that feel good and do them every day. If you faithfully and consistently practice them as I've described, you should begin to feel a difference within two weeks.

A huge percentage of the U.S. population has lower back muscles that are overtightened, overstressed, and overworked because of the weakened midback muscles that do not perform the way they were meant to. This program strengthens *all* the muscles in the back and can alleviate that problem.

Regardless of how you use the program, the secret to success is to use it. Don't let this be just another book of exercises that sits on your shelf as you become more and more discouraged about constant back pain or your appearance. If you do the program, it will work!

Getting in Touch

An alternative form of healing and rejuvenation that has made a fabulous comeback is massage. I highly recommend that you find yourself a good massage, neuromuscular, or sports massage therapist, or any credentialed professional who specializes in what is known as "soft tissue" work. Some specialize in techniques used to relieve specific injuries and conditions, while others work to release blocked energy and to clear toxins from the body, providing an overall sense of relaxation and well-being.

In order for these exercises to achieve maximum results (and they can improve your posture and relieve your pain), the muscles and underlying tissues must be healthy. That's where massage comes in. Beginning a treatment program of weekly massage as you start the exercises will greatly speed your progress. As you begin to see and feel the changes in your body you can cut back to massage therapy once every two weeks.

Begin to practice the art of conscious breathing and purposeful movement. We live in our bodies and yet take them completely for granted. Once a day, stop and notice what you are feeling. See if you can identify tension or fatigue or discomfort. The skill of feeling our physicalness, the awareness of sensation in the body, is part of what tells us we are alive, and it allows us to identify physical stress in the body before it becomes chronic. This program is a key to making some powerful changes in your life. These are not just exercises, they are a whole new way of being in your body.

BIBLIOGRAPHY

Alter, Michael J. 1988. *Science of Stretching.* Champaign, Ill.: Human Kinetics.

Ammer, Christine. 1992. *Have a Nice Day—No Problem.* New York: Penguin Books.

Bland, John H. 1987. *Disorders of the Cervical Spine, 2nd Ed.* Philadelphia: W. B. Saunders.

Boden, Scott D., Sam W. Wiesel, Edward R. Laws, Richard H. Rothman. 1991. *The Aging Spine: Essentials of Pathophysiology, Diagnosis and Treatment.* Philadelphia: W. B. Saunders.

Bohannon, Richard W. 1991–1992. *Journal of Human Muscle Performance.*

Brunstrom, Signe. 1975. *Clinical Kinesiology, 3rd Ed.* Revised by Ruth Dickinson. Philadelphia: F. A. Davis Co.

Calais-Germain, Blandine. 1993. *Anatomy of Movement.* Seattle: Eastland Press.

Cantu, Robert I., and Alan J. Grodin. 1992. *Myofascial Manipulation: Theory and Clinical Application.* Gaithersburg, Md.: Aspen Publishers.

Christensen, Alice, and David Rankin. 1975. *Easy Does It Yoga.* New York: Harper & Row.

Daniels, Lucille, and Catherine Worthingham. 1977. *Therapeutic Exercise, 2nd Ed.* Philadelphia: W. B. Saunders.

Hanna, Thomas. 1988. *Somatics.* Reading, Mass.: Addison-Wesley.

Jenkins, David B. 1991. *Hollinshead's Functional Anatomy of the Limbs and Back, 6th Ed.* Philadelphia: W. B. Saunders.

Kabat-Zinn, Jon. 1990. *Full Catastrophe Living: Using the Wisdom of Your Body and Mind to Face Stress, Pain and Illness.* New York: Bantam Doubleday Dell, Delta Books.

Kendall, Florence P., and Elizabeth Kendall McCreary. 1993. *Muscles: Testing and Function. 4th Ed.* Baltimore: Williams and Wilkins.

Kendall, Henry O., Florence P. Kendall, and Dorothy A. Boynton. 1981. *Posture and Pain.* Baltimore: Williams and Wilkins.

Le Veau, Barney F. 1992. *Williams and Lissner's Biomechanics of Human Motion, 3rd Ed.* Philadephia: W. B. Saunders.

Mattes, Aaron L. 1990. *Flexibility, Active and Assisted Stretching.* Sarasota, Fla.: Aaron L. Mattes.

McAtee, Robert E. 1993. *Facilitated Stretching.* Champaign, Ill.: Human Kinetics.

Mennel, John McM. 1992. *The Musculoskeletal System: Differential Diagnosis from Symptoms and Physical Signs.* Gaithersburg, Md.: Aspen Publishers.

Pheasant, Stephen. 1991. *Ergonomics, Work and Health.* Gaithersburg, Md.: Aspen Publishers.

Schatz, Mary Pullig. 1992. *Back Care Basics.* Berkeley, Calif.: Rodmell Press.

Sieg, Kay W., and Sandra P. Adams. 1992. *Illustrated Essentials of Musculoskeletal Anatomy, 2nd Ed.* Gainesville, Fla.: Mega Books.

Breathworks Audio Tapes
with Nancy Swayzee

To order tapes of the exercises in Breathworks, fill out the form at the bottom of the page.

Breathworks . . . Strengthening Your Back
From the Inside Out Tape I
Phenomenal Abdominals Program 90 minutes

This tape leads you progressively through the abdominal strengthening program. The tape is divided into two 45-minute segments. Basic and intermediate exercises are on one side, advanced exercises on the other. Both sides begin with belly breathing and guided visualization to allow you to enter a state of deep relaxation and body awareness. The two 45-minute sides are spaced so that you may do as few or as many exercises as you choose.

Breathworks . . . Strengthening Your Back
From the Inside Out Tape II
Within Range and Back to Back Basics 90 minutes

This one-hour tape has range of motion exercises on one side and the back strengthening program and moving stretches on the other. The range-of-motion exercises serve as either a warmup for the back strengthening program or as gentle strengthening exercises for someone recovering from an injury or surgery. Both sides begin with belly breathing and guided visualization to allow you to enter a state of deep relaxation and body awareness. The two 45-minute sides are spaced so that you may do as few or as many exercises as you choose.

Send order blank to C.E.T. For Life Exercise Therapy
P.O. Box 877
Cedar Ridge, CA 95924
- -

2 Tape Set $10.95
Please send me: __ set(s) of Tape I & Tape II
Add $1.00 for postage and handling
Calif. residents add 7.25% tax
Total _____
Make checks payable to C.E.T. For Life